What fellow Reiki Masters had to say about

Reiki for the Heart and Soul

"Amy Rowland elegantly and eloquently shares how we may each 'walk our talk' by offering riveting, real-life examples of how present-day Reiki Masters and esteemed Reiki Masters of the past have utilized, and continue to utilize, the Reiki principles in a dynamic and living way, every day. This is a must read for humanity!"

Sensei John King, R.M., D.D., author of
Breathology: How To Breathe Yourself To Better Health

"This is a well-written Reiki book that weaves together many important details with a wonderful spiritual sentiment. It grounds one in the here and now and inspires practitioners to look deeply into their own healing and to help others."

William Lee Rand, author of *Reiki: The Healing Touch* and
director of the International Center for Reiki Training

"A joyful read! Amy Rowland provides a heartfelt guide for living Reiki in our daily lives. This book will help you open to Reiki as a spiritual path."

Carolyn Musial, teacher/practitioner with the
International Center for Reiki Training and author of
Communicating with Animals: A Presentation & Meditation

"Amy Rowland has once again written an invaluable and insightful book. *Reiki for the Heart and Soul* not only provides an excellent overview of the Reiki system but also explores, for the first time, the Reiki principles from a place of depth and authenticity. This book exemplifies the very essence of Reiki and provides us with a map of how we can genuinely use these teachings for the betterment of ourselves and humanity."

Lawrence Ellyard, author of *Reiki: 200 Questions and*
Answers for Beginners* and *Reiki Meditations for Beginners

"An in-depth book on the principles of Reiki and mindfulness of their values—recommended both to newcomers and established practitioners."

Tanmaya Honervogt, author of *The Power of Reiki:*
An Ancient Hands-On Healing Technique

REIKI
for the Heart and Soul

The Reiki Principles
as
Spiritual Pathwork

AMY Z. ROWLAND

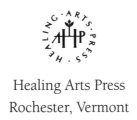

Healing Arts Press
Rochester, Vermont

Healing Arts Press
One Park Street
Rochester, Vermont 05767
www.HealingArtsPress.com

Healing Arts Press is a division of Inner Traditions International

Note to the reader: *This book is intended as an informational guide. The remedies, approaches, and techniques described herein are meant to supplement, and not to be a substitute for, professional medical care or treatment. They should not be used to treat a serious ailment without prior consultation with a qualified health care professional.*

Library of Congress Cataloging-in-Publication Data

Rowland, Amy Zaffarano.
  Reiki for the heart and soul : the Reiki principles as spiritual pathwork / Amy Z. Rowland.
      p. cm.
  Includes bibliographical references.
   Summary: "How the principles of Reiki can be used not just for healing but also for spiritual growth"—Provided by publisher.
  ISBN 978-1-59477-252-8 (pbk.)
 1. Spiritual life. 2. Reiki (Healing system) I. Title.
  BL624.R69 2008
  131—dc22
                                                                                    2008032781

Printed and bound in Canada by Transcontinental Printing

10   9   8   7   6   5   4   3   2   1

Text design and layout by Virginia Scott Bowman
This book was typeset in Berkeley Oldstyle with Amadeus and Eve as display typefaces

Photographs of Lauren Bissett and Albert Seaman by Connie Bell-Dixon.
Page 46: Image of the Gainen, inscribed by Dave King, used with his permission.

To send correspondence to the author of this book, mail a first-class letter to the author c/o Inner Traditions • Bear & Company, One Park Street, Rochester, VT 05767, and we will forward the communication. For more information on her books and work or how to contact her directly, please visit her website at **www.traditionalreiki.com.**

To you, who read this book with hope:
may it light the way ahead
and show you the next few steps
you might take on your path
"just for today . . ."

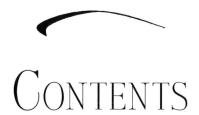

CONTENTS

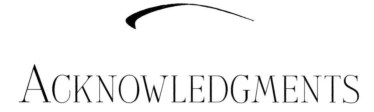

ACKNOWLEDGMENTS

This book begins and ends in gratitude, which centers me and steadies me and enables me to go forward on my life's path. I am grateful to be alive on the planet Earth at this challenging time, to have a loving family and good friends, and to have encountered so many helpful strangers and pleasant "traveling companions" on my life's journey to this point. I am also grateful for the journey itself, with all its ups and downs, and twists and turns. I have learned from this adventure, from the marvels and wonders, the crises, and the periods of calm—and I am still learning. For this opportunity, I am grateful to Spirit.

No words can describe fully how Reiki has changed me and continues to change me, healing so much in me that I thought could not be healed, bringing me greater peace and contentment than I thought possible. I am grateful to my teachers: Reiki Masters Beth Gray and Frank DuGan who taught me Usui Shiki Ryoho Reiki, and to the teachers who came before them: Hawayo Takata, Chujiro Hayashi, and Mikao Usui. I also deeply value the teachings of Usui Reiki Ryoho, which I learned from Tom Rigler, Hiroshi Doi, and Hyakuten Inamoto, and I am pleased to have learned Gendai and Komyo Reiki, modern forms that blend the two traditions so well. I revere those who have attempted to gain a clearer understanding of Reiki's early origins in Japan and who have generously shared what they have learned; and I am grateful to every translator who has helped in this scholarly task. I am so glad to know more about the lives of Hawayo Takata and Chujiro Hayashi through the stories that have been passed down by the twenty-two Reiki masters she trained, and I have delighted in reading accounts of Mrs. Takata's life in the books by Fran Brown, Helen

Haberly, and Annali Twan, and in hearing Mrs. Takata's voice on the audiocassette made available by John Harvey Gray. I also appreciate the ongoing support of the Reiki world community offered by William Lee Rand and the many other Reiki masters who write about Reiki in books and in magazine articles. Thank you all!

Even closer to my heart are those who have honored me by choosing me as a teacher or practitioner. It has been my privilege to share in the Reiki energy with you for an hour or two, or a day or two, or years. For however long we have come together with the purpose of learning more about Reiki healing, I am grateful. Donna Davidson and Scott Pruyn, proprietors of the Dreamcatcher (www.dreamcatcherweb.com) in Skippack, Pennsylvania, thank you for providing a wonderful space for so many Reiki classes and Reikishares, and for your wisdom, kindness, and love of Reiki.

My thanks to all who agreed to share stories of your experiences in practicing Reiki energy healing and attempting to live by the Reiki principles: Karen Biehl; Lauren Bissett; Jim and Linda Chokas; Kenneth Donnelly: Raymond Feist; Barbara Friling; Terry and John Graybill; Paula Heller; Ian Meinzer; Aimee Kovac; Leslie Levy; Alexis McVeigh; Ikechukwu Omenka; Ellen Phillips; Sharon and Rick Riegner; Tina Roach; Bob Rowlands; Noreen Ryen and Bryan Benford; Lauren Sage; Barbara Sautter; Beverly Schultz; Al Seaman; Michael Sebio; Connie Seneko; Kay, Jim, and Paul Sivel; Judi Taylor; Karen Thompson; Linda Urie; Charlie Wagg; Janny Wurts; Iryna Zhyrenko; as well as those who asked not to be identified by name. Your kindness in sharing your stories lights the way ahead, the goodness of your hearts gives comfort, and the strength of your courage inspires others.

Lauren Bissett and Al Seaman, thank you for agreeing to be the models for the photographs in this book. You are so beautiful to me. I see the light of your souls whenever I look into your eyes. I believe that readers will see it, too. Connie Bell-Dixon, it is good to work with a photographer who is so professional and easygoing, and who loves Reiki. I appreciate your work—and your friendship.

For dedication, for healing, and for understanding, I extend my deepest thanks to all the members of the distant-healing list e-mail group. Sharon Riegner, Eileen Morgan, and Betsy Ingram, thank you for the hands-on Reiki sessions—and for your compassionate care. David Gleekel, my thanks to you as well for Reiki sessions and distant healing that rested and relaxed and healed me when I felt most under stress.

And David, what can I say? Thank you for channeling Mrs. Takata one fine spring day last year to tell me that I was going to write another book "on the Reiki principles—and more." Steve Ritch, thank you for making all my stays in Washington with you feel like I'm coming home. All my students in Washington, DC, through the Reiki Center of Greater Washington, thank you for your support and friendship. You expand my world.

Jon Graham, acquisitions editor at Inner Traditions • Bear & Company, I am grateful to you for agreeing to my proposal for this book with lightning speed, counter to all my expectations of the publishing world. Ehud Sperling, Kelly Bowen, Jeanie Levitan, Cynthia Fowles, Andy Raymond, Jessica Arsenault, Manzanita Carpenter, and everyone else at Inner Traditions • Bear & Company, I appreciate everything you do to keep your authors happy and our books in print and available worldwide. I am so glad to be one of them! Jamaica Burns, thank you for your patience, your hard work, your gentle approach to working with me as an author. You have made this a better book.

How could I ever get through a book without the special hand-holding of my writing buddies? Ellen Phillips, I respect you so much as a fellow Reiki master and value you so much as a friend that the fact that you are a top-notch freelance editor and writer often slips my mind—until I have a publishing question! Thank you for all your sound advice. Donna Fasano, in phone call after phone call, you never judge me and tell me that I could have done better; instead, you are kind and caring, making it so much easier to sit down again at the keyboard and start writing. Fred Even, you treat me to a wonderful dinner and talk writing with me, month after month. It matters so much that you believe in me. My dear friend Mark Clutton, who wrote to me from the United Kingdom to say that you liked *Intuitive Reiki for Our Times* and then just kept writing, what a delight it is to know you. Thank you for your encouragement—and for the chocolate, the beautiful skeins of yarn from the Isle of Skye, and so many entertaining transatlantic conversations.

Finally, I thank you who hold this book in your hands. As you read these acknowledgments, may you be reminded of the chance encounters and the enduring friendships that have made your life's journey worthwhile; and as you read on, may you recall those who have helped you understand more about the nature of peace, taught you something about integrity, and touched your life with kindness. Join with me in feeling gratitude—and let's go forward, hand in hand, in grace and in the spirit of Reiki healing.

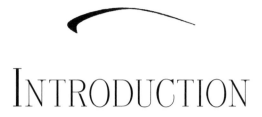

INTRODUCTION

One day a few years ago, I awoke with the realization that I dreaded the day. There had been several deaths in the family, as well as some legal and financial difficulties. Although the latter didn't directly affect me, I still felt anxious for those I loved. Negative thoughts darted through my mind like birds confined in a cage as my feelings moved between weariness, sorrow, and worry.

As I became more awake, I remembered the recent translations of the Reiki principles, which Mikao Usui had boldly titled "The Secret Method of Inviting Happiness/The Miracle Medicine for All Diseases." Did he mean that the practice of Reiki energy healing invited happiness, or was he recommending the recitation and application of the principles as a way to greater well-being? I practiced Reiki every day. If I wasn't happy, then he couldn't mean that Reiki energy healing alone was the route to happiness, could he? If so, why did I seem so far off track?

So I began to reflect on the Reiki principles each day, noting my thoughts in my journal and asking myself how I was applying each principle in my own life. I also pondered the relationship between the energy and the principles. By giving the original principles a double title, Mikao Usui had somehow intertwined the practice of energy healing with his recommendation to recite the principles each day, morning and night. Defying my Western mindset, I began to say the principles to myself before I did Reiki in the morning, and as I lay in bed at night doing hands-on Reiki and drifting off to sleep.

One morning, with a jolt of surprise, I realized that just as Reiki energy healing is intended to be used not only on others but also on ourselves, so the Reiki principles are intended to be applied not only in our relationships, but also in our individual lives. It doesn't do much good to avoid becoming angry with others if we often feel frustrated and annoyed with ourselves. It's not effective to set aside today's worries over work or love if we allow thoughts about illnesses we may suffer in old age to drift through our minds all day. It's good to be grateful for the blessings that come to us through others, but what about being grateful for our own lives, and for the talents and skills we have that enable us to make a contribution in the world? Doing an honest day's work is a fine intention, but what's an honest day's work on a Saturday or Sunday, when most people normally take time off? How do we find the balance between doing too much and too little? It's easy to understand how we can be kind to others, but how can we be kind to ourselves? What's the difference between reciting the principles and remembering the principles? Is remembrance the same as mindfulness?

I realized that I had stumbled onto a Pandora's box of questions that seemed to have no answers—or none that I understood at the time. And if I, with many years of experience practicing and teaching Reiki, felt confused, then how did less experienced Reiki practitioners and teachers feel? The issue of the place of the Reiki principles in practice seemed worth exploring, and it seemed likely that the results would be worth sharing. Like a hiker determined to make good time during daylight, I set out and soon realized that I was engaged in spiritual pathwork: discovering how practicing Reiki energy healing and its principles together advance the journey of the soul.

This awareness made me recall an actual journey that I had taken years ago. Late one summer afternoon, I set off to walk down a country road and into a wilderness refuge—but my journey went awry. Without adequate knowledge of the territory I was exploring, without proper equipment or any provisions, I was unable to complete the route I had planned before darkness fell. I ended up scratched, wet, hungry, and frustrated because I had to retrace my steps in order to get out of the woods before nightfall. When I reached home, I discovered that I had been gone five hours, but I might as well have been gone five years. My journey had changed me. I had almost gotten lost, but I had also found a new appreciation for the value of "traveling companions." I felt particularly grateful to my Reiki friends, who walked the path of Reiki with me, and who, from time to time, shared their stories and shined the light of wisdom on the way ahead.

This book gives you the opportunity to connect with others who walk the path of Reiki to help you understand that many have traveled the path before you and succeeded in achieving greater health, well-being, and happiness. Think of the individual practitioners and teachers whose stories you read here as traveling companions. They may remind you of the value of moral decisiveness, offer another perspective that helps you to recognize crisis as an opportunity for growth, or inspire you to have greater courage in the face of difficulty.

It is my hope that after reflecting on the stories and considering some of the suggestions for deepening practice, you will feel inspired to apply the principles more often in your own life. It's not always easy to walk away from anger, to set aside preoccupation with worry, to be grateful for life just as it is, to be honest and honorable, or to be kind. Yet those who make the effort to do so—to accept the Reiki principles as guidance for achieving a better way of life—are rewarded with peace of mind, contentment, and a sense of personal integrity that are to be valued as much as any spiritual treasures.

This book begins by describing some experiences common to new Reiki practitioners, which may become the foundation for a deeper spiritual understanding. How is this understanding reflected in the Reiki principles, in their many translations? Each principle is considered worthy of contemplation in its own right and is given a separate chapter, as are the twin titles given to the principles by Mikao Usui. Each chapter contains some suggested Reiki techniques to support you in incorporating the principles; some suggestions for meditation and reflection; and other exercises that may help you heal, better understand yourself, integrate self-knowledge, claim empowerment, and discover peace of mind and happiness. The book concludes with an invitation to look at practice of the principles as spiritual pathwork, which requires persistence, patience, and daily commitment.

For those who learned Reiki in the Western tradition, Usui Shiki Ryoho, the principles are a bit like five small, rough diamonds given to us at the start of a journey; we're told not to worry about them, put them in a back pocket, go on our way, and practice Reiki healing daily. For practitioners who learned

Reiki in Japan, through the Usui Reiki Ryoho Gakkai, the principles hold a far more important place, for the complete principles, with titles and the founder's recommendation, are widely known. Reiki practitioners are encouraged to recite the principles, morning and night, to foster mindfulness throughout the day.

So check your back pocket. Are those five rough diamonds still tucked safely away there? Dig them out. Hold them in your hand. Think about what they're worth to you right now. Think about what they might be worth to you tumbled and polished. It's up to you to do the spiritual work, to look at the principles and recognize their value in your life, to consider them until you have a refined understanding of how they help you to heal yourself and to bring others greater healing through Reiki. This is the prospect that opens before you: a clearer path to miracles—and to happiness.

Thank you for joining me on this journey.

1

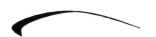

THE PATH OF REIKI

When Mikao Usui climbed Mt. Kurama with the intention of meditating, fasting, and praying for twenty-one days in the hope of achieving wisdom, he did not know if he would survive. He did not know if he would ever make the return journey to the city of Kyoto. He did not know if he would ever again see family, friends, or professional colleagues. He set aside all these worldly concerns and climbed the mountain, going slowly where the way was difficult and steep, walking steadily where the way was clear. Perhaps he encountered obstructions—a fallen tree that forced him to bend beneath its branches or a stream swollen with spring rain that required him to make slight changes in his course. Still he remained focused on his purpose and completed his journey.

According to traditional Japanese Reiki teachings, Usui climbed Mt. Kurama in pursuit of enlightenment. Those teaching in the Western (Usui Shiki Ryoho) tradition say that Usui journeyed up the mountain to seek guidance regarding reintroducing the world to Reiki, an ancient laying-on-of-hands healing method he had long sought and finally found described on a dusty, forgotten scroll in the archives of a temple library in Kyoto. Whatever his actual purpose, both Eastern and Western traditions agree that at the end of the twenty-one days, Mikao Usui experienced a profound spiritual event, a spontaneous initiation that transformed his limited awareness and understanding into complete consciousness of the energy that would later be called Reiki. This experience of the energy also healed him of all weakness from his long fast and energized him so that he leaped to his feet and took off running down the mountain.

Both accounts also record that Usui first used Reiki on himself. In his great hurry to descend the mountain and return to Kyoto to share with others what he had experienced, he ran down the trail. Almost as soon as he had begun, he tripped over a stone and tore the skin and nail of his big toe. He did what anyone would do: he stopped running and bent down to inspect his injury; then he cupped his hands around the throbbing toe to give himself the comfort of touch. Of course, his touch had been transformed by his spontaneous attunement to the energy. Within a very short time, the bleeding stopped and the pain was gone, and when he looked at the toe again, he saw that the broken skin was healed. It was as if the injury had never been. Reflecting on this miracle, Usui returned to the path, now walking at a comfortable pace.

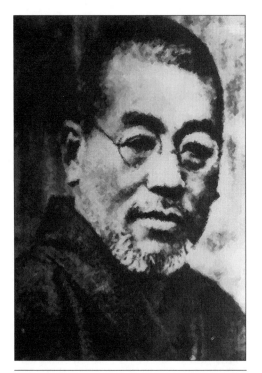

Charcoal rendering of the familiar photo of Mikao Usui

Reiki historians say that Mikao Usui's journey up Mt. Kurama; his twenty-one-day meditation, fast, and prayer vigil; and his attunement to the Reiki energy took place in March 1922. This was a real journey: the ascent of a sacred mountain to its peak and the spiritual experience of a lifetime, followed by the descent of the same mountain and the continuation of that lifetime in spiritual service.

Anyone who has ever attempted to achieve a worthy goal and met challenges and hardships before achieving success can appreciate the story of this journey, and every human being who has recognized life as a journey of growth and transformation can understand it. For Reiki practitioners and teachers, it's easy to see these parallels and draw inspiration from the story. For many of us, just as for Mikao Usui, the journey to Reiki is not an easy one. However, attunement to Reiki marks a life-changing moment for us all, and our experience of that first miracle of healing gives us reason to slow down, pause, and reflect.

STARTING FROM WHEREVER YOU ARE

People come to Reiki in many ways. There is no one right way to "enter" onto the path. Many people are inspired to learn Reiki when they experience its benefits at the hands of a friend who is a practitioner and able to provide quick relief from headache or sore throat or tired, tense shoulders. Others decide to learn Reiki when they see how effectively it brings comfort and deep relaxation to someone they love who has become seriously ill. This desire to bring relief from pain, to offer comfort, and to speed healing is easy to understand.

Yet people come to Reiki for many other reasons as well. Some find that they enjoy exploring alternative healing and discover Reiki somewhere between aromatherapy and Vogel crystals. Some people recognize that the religion of their childhood no longer satisfies them spiritually, and they turn to Reiki, hoping for a stronger sense of connection to God. Others claim curiosity brings them to Reiki I class, nothing more.

Whatever our life journeys have been, however prepared or unprepared we feel before we learn Reiki, we must start from where we are. We must accept the circumstances that have brought us to the point where we sit in a chair, waiting to be attuned to the Reiki energy. Our level of education doesn't matter. Our religious background doesn't matter. Our training or lack of training in healthcare or an allied field doesn't matter. Our age, gender, race, and ethnic background do not matter. We may be intuitive and insightful, or we may be innocent and naïve. We must start from where we are, aware—or unaware—of all our limitations and imperfections, in order to go forward on the path of Reiki healing and to become whole.

ONE BEGINNING

A few years ago, I opened my e-mail to read this message from a prospective Reiki student named Lauren Bissett:

> Greetings! I have been interested in Reiki for several years but have yet to study or experience its teachings. I recently learned of the classes you teach at Dreamcatcher. Although I hope to take a class, I am also interested in receiving treatment. Are there sessions available to those in search of Reiki treatment? If you have more information, I would greatly appreciate it.
>
> I hope to accelerate my burn recovery. Five months ago, I experienced second and third degree burns to my face, hands, and upper arm. My burns were treated with a bioengineered skin, which accelerated the healing, reducing scarring. However, my chin and an area on my arm did not take to the surgery. These wounds took over a month to heal, which left me with twelve to eighteen months of scar management . . . I am fighting raised hypertrophic scarring, which has the potential to grow up to a half inch, with uncomfortable pressure garments, silicon sheeting, and so on. My scars are causing me increasing discomfort, and I am hoping to accelerate the healing process. I am only five months out, and I cannot imagine my daily rituals of scar management continuing for another seven or more months. It has been so consuming.
>
> Recently, I have read incredible testimonies by burn survivors who were treated with Reiki, which has increased my interest in Reiki and your practice. I have ordered *Traditional Reiki for Our Times,* and anxiously anticipate reading your work! Thank you so much for your time and for sharing Reiki in Skippack. I look forward to hearing from you![1]

Lauren had taken a digital photo of herself that she sent as an attachment with her e-mail. The image astonished me: it showed only part of her face. Her dark-brown eyes, straight nose, and full mouth were framed like a window by the white pressure garment. Most of her head, neck, and arms were encased in bandages. She looked like a partially wrapped mummy! Her eyes shone brightly, and I could "read" in them both sadness and the smallest spark of hope.

What had happened? How had she sustained such injuries? I wrote back to her immediately and offered to do a Reiki treatment in the privacy of her home; and if she would like, at a later time I would teach her Reiki one on one in the same setting. Her reply was immediate. She would greatly appreciate that courtesy, because proper burn care meant that she could not go out in the sun at all. Her skin was still far too sensitive. Within a few days, we spoke on the phone and scheduled an appointment for a complete Reiki treatment. During the session, she felt deeply relaxed. She later told me that she had slept well that night for the first time since she had sustained the burn injuries. The confinement of the pressure garment, the smell and feel of the salve she had to apply, and even the itchiness of her healing skin had not bothered her. "That was the best night's sleep of my life!" she exclaimed. "I want to learn Reiki."

During her Reiki I class, Lauren told me that since the burn accident, she had felt at loose ends, unable to attend art school or work and confined to her apartment most of the time to protect her healing skin from sun damage. Though unsure what she would do next, she was very glad to learn Reiki, and she was intrigued by the process of learning to "listen" to the Reiki energy flowing through her hands. After the class, Lauren did a lot of Reiki on herself, day and night, to speed her own recovery and to make the long process of healing more comfortable. She did wear a pressure garment on her face and neck for about a year and a half, but she found that she could endure the discomfort with good humor, and her skin healed remarkably well.

This interval of time was healing in another way: as Lauren continued to receive outpatient burn care and to do Reiki, she realized that her own career interests were changing. She decided that when she was well enough to go out again, rather than returning to art school, she would enroll in a nursing program at a nearby community college as a first step toward become a registered nurse (RN) specializing in burn care. She would also continue to study Reiki.

How successful has she been in realizing her dream? Lauren's recovery from her own burn injuries is complete; she is the female model for this book.

In May 2008, she graduated from community college, was certified as a registered nurse, and welcomed on staff at a local hospital. She has continued with her Reiki training, through the advanced course and the master course, and she will very soon be certified to teach Reiki.

LEARNING TO LISTEN TO THE ENERGY

In a traditionally taught Reiki class in the Western (Usui Shiki Ryoho) tradition, the teacher emphasizes the importance of learning to listen to the Reiki energy as it flows through the hands to bring healing. Often, before a class, some students will notice sensations of warmth or tingling "visiting" them; the energy is already on its way, special delivery! Of course, this is just a sample of the many sensations and the expanded perception that come with the experience of the Reiki attunement.

When I teach Reiki I, I reassure students that whatever happens during the attunements is okay. If they find themselves enjoying a sense of peace, noticing a pulsing in their fingertips, or surprised by a swirl of purple color visible to them with closed eyes, this is fine. And if they feel nothing different or remarkable, this, too, is just fine. As the attunements are repeated throughout the class, almost all students feel some sensations of the energy, but those who don't will grow into that awareness through hands-on practice.

How do we learn to listen to the energy? During a traditional class, most Reiki teachers will describe some of the sensations that the students might perceive. These range from mild warmth to intense heat, and coolness to icy cold. Besides differences in temperature, practitioners often notice tingling. This, too, may be very light or quite strong. Sometimes practitioners describe feeling a hum of current, remarkably like the low vibration of a small appliance, such as a radio, plugged into an electrical outlet but with the power off. Other words sometimes used to describe the sensations of energy are "buzzing," "bubbling," "pins and needles but without any pain." Some practitioners report feeling pulsing, whirls, or waves of energy. Others notice a sense of pressure or magnetism that seems to hold their hands in place.

Through practicing a complete client treatment, all students in a traditionally taught Reiki I class are given the opportunity to begin training their attention on the flow of the energy. Besides noticing the subtle sensations in their hands, they're also asked to notice the increases and decreases in activity to determine when to move their hands to the next standard position.*

In Japan as well, traditionally taught (Usui Reiki Ryoho) practitioners who have practiced basic hand positions and demonstrated a basic understanding are invited to learn Byosen Reikan-ho, or scanning of the energy field around the client's body. This requires that they learn to notice (or "listen" to) the sensations in their hands, called *hibiki,* or "resonance." They're told that these sensations will occur over any area of the body where there is illness or injury, stress or tension—a sign of disruption in the energy flow. Mastery of Byosen Reikan-ho and one other technique, called Reiji-ho, are required to advance to the next level. Reiji-ho is another way of listening to the Reiki energy; using this technique, practitioners ask for guidance throughout the treatment regarding hand placement until the treatment is complete.†

NOW YOU:
PRACTICE LISTENING TO THE ENERGY

How can practitioners improve their ability to listen to the energy? Besides focusing on the energy during hands-on healing, whether in self-treatment or client-treatment, there is a wonderful meditation that has been taught in the Usui Reiki Ryoho Gakkai (the Japanese Reiki learning society). Historically, this technique has been taught at the Shoden (entry) and Okuden (deep mystery) levels of Usui Reiki Ryoho training. The meditation, called Hatsurei-ho, may be entered into at any moment, once mastered. However, to begin learning the meditation, it's good to adopt the same ritual gestures that have been used in the past by Japanese

---

*For more about this technique of "listening to the energy," please see my book *Traditional Reiki for Our Times: Practical Methods for Personal and Planetary Healing,* which is noted in Recommended Reading and Listening along with other titles referenced in the text.

†The basis of my understanding of these traditional Japanese techniques is practice and instruction. In addition to being trained in Usui Shiki Ryoho Reiki I and II in 1987 with Beth Gray, and Reiki III in 1994 with Frank DuGan, I was trained in the Usui Reiki Ryoho tradition in 2001 and Gendai Reiki (modern Reiki) in 2002 by Tom Rigler. In September of the same year, I attended the Usui Reiki Ryoho International Workshop, where I had the opportunity to meet Mr. Hiroshi Doi in person to review Usui Reiki Ryoho and Gendai techniques, and to receive additional instruction.

Reiki practitioners and teachers. It's also good to sit down in a sturdy chair that allows you to place your feet flat on the ground and that supports your back so that your spine is relatively straight, allowing you to breathe deeply. When you're comfortable with the gestures, the focused intention, and the breathing, and familiar with the effects of this meditation, you may want to try performing it sitting or kneeling on the floor or standing erect.

1. In a comfortable, relaxed posture, with your hands resting palms down on your thighs, set your intention to do Hatsurei-ho. This is a meditation on the Reiki energy that will help to clear away any negativity that you feel and also help you become more aware of the Reiki energy in your hands and elsewhere in your body, because it intensifies sensations of the energy.

2. Perform Kenyoku-ho, or Dry Brushing. With your right hand, fingers extended, but relaxed, reach up to your left shoulder and quickly sweep down and across your chest (fig. 1.1). Complete the motion by allowing your right arm to return to a relaxed, comfortable position at your side. Do the same with your left hand, reaching up to your right shoulder (fig. 1.2) and quickly sweeping down and across your chest (fig. 1.3). Once more, with your right hand, reach up to your left shoulder and quickly sweep down and across your chest.

   Then use your right hand, with fingers extended, to quickly sweep down your left arm, from shoulder to palm (fig. 1.4). Repeat this gesture with your left hand on your right arm (fig. 1.5); and then, once more, with your right hand on your left arm (fig. 1.6).[2] (If you find it more comfortable to do so, you may repeat these three motions from elbow to palm, rather than shoulder to palm. Both are acceptable.) Although this ritual may seem awkward at first, it is easy to learn to perform it very quickly, as the Japanese do.

3. Lift up your arms toward the sky so that your hands reach for the Reiki energy that flows into you from above (see fig. 1.7 on page 15). Breathe with awareness of this flow. Visualize or imagine the Reiki energy as light descending from above, filling you, and surrounding you so that you're within a column of light.

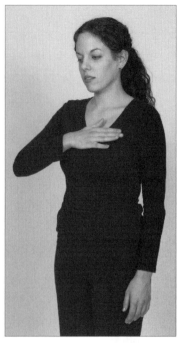

Figure 1.1

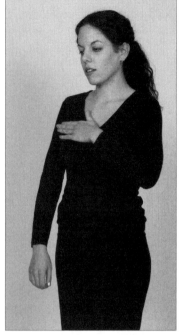

Figure 1.2

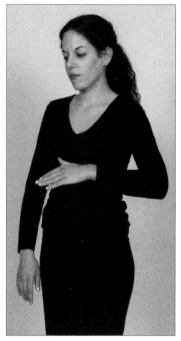

Figure 1.3

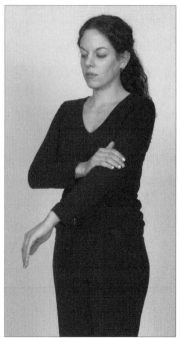

Figure 1.4

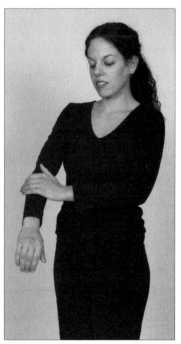

Figure 1.5

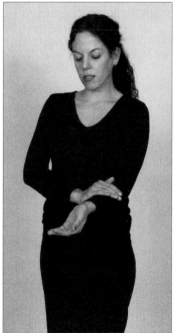

Figure 1.6

4. Breathe slowly and relax, enjoying any sensations of the energy that you notice in your hands, your feet, and elsewhere in your body. This is Joshin Koku ho or "cleansing breathing," which quiets and clears the mind.

5. Perform *gassho:* bring your hands together palm to palm (fig. 1.8), in the universal gesture of prayer and meditation; allow your mind to become quiet.

If it seems too difficult to find stillness within, you may try this technique, called Sei Shin Totsu, or Concentration, which is recommended by Mr. Hiroshi Doi:

6. As you breathe in the Reiki energy through the crown of your head and your nose, notice the path that it travels down through your windpipe, filling your lungs. Notice that it travels down even farther, following the column of your spine all the way into your belly. Let it concentrate there, a few centimeters below the navel, at the point the Japanese call the *tan-den.* Breathe in and out slowly, noticing the energy flowing into you with each inhalation, concentrating at the tan-den, and then releasing into your energy field with each exhalation.

7. Imagine that you can breathe in the Reiki energy through your hands. Inhale, breathing in Reiki through your hands, your nose, and the crown of your head. Let it concentrate for a few seconds in your tan-den. Then breathe out, radiating Reiki through your hands and your whole being. (You may want to make a sound as you breathe out, a long "ah" of release. This is called *hado* breathing, and you may find that it enhances the meditation. See chapter 4 for detailed information on hado breathing.) Remain focused on the flow of the Reiki energy, breathing it in and out through your hands for a few minutes. Listen to the energy everywhere in and around you.

8. Conclude the meditation whenever it feels appropriate, with an acknowledgment that you are finishing Hatsurei-ho. You may wish to bow to the energy that has cleansed you, brought you healing, and bathed you in light before shaking out your hands and letting them come to rest again in your lap (fig. 1.9).[3]

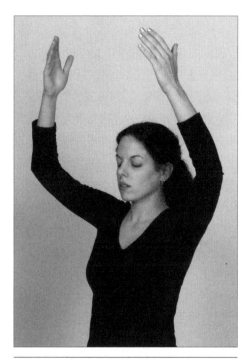

Figure 1.7

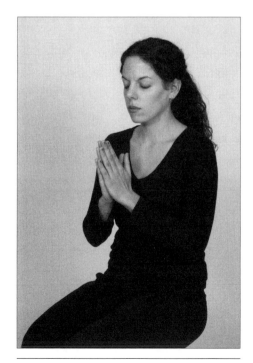

Figure 1.8

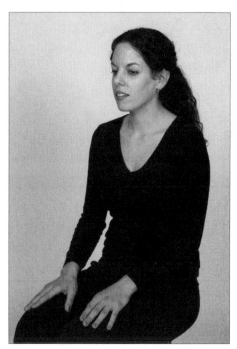

Figure 1.9

As we learn to listen to the Reiki energy, we gradually become more conscious of its source in Spirit. Just as when we follow a stream to where it first emerges from the ground as a trickle of springwater or a tumble of waterfall, we may feel child-like joy in this discovery, and we may realize that we feel refreshed and renewed. We take in what we're meant to take in, almost without effort, and we're restored to an awareness of essential nature. In this way, the gentle practice of "listening to the energy" may offer us benefits like those of more formal meditations.

In Japan, meditating on the energy, using Hatsurei-ho or similar techniques, is a common practice, but traditional Reiki practitioners also recite the Reiki principles with mindfulness twice each day, morning and night, as Mikao Usui recommended to his students. In the West, the Reiki principles have been presented for decades without this recommendation. The Reiki master's encouragement to meditate on the principles is often a very mild one.

It's up to each of us as individuals to decide how much time and energy we want to give to Reiki practice, how much we want to deepen our knowledge of its history, and to what extent we want to focus on becoming better acquainted with the energy through daily self-treatment, client treatment, and meditation. It's a pleasure to learn to listen to the energy, however. Once we make this discovery, we find ways to make more room for Reiki in our lives: we get up a half hour earlier to do hands-on healing on ourselves; we buy a book about Reiki's history and read it in spare moments; we establish a quiet time after work when we can send distant healing. We pursue our interest in Reiki at our own speed, even if that speed satisfies no one but ourselves—and that is wonderful.

GOING FORWARD AT YOUR OWN PACE

Sometimes inner guidance prompts us to move forward even before we've agreed to the destination. In *Intuitive Reiki for Our Times: Essential Techniques for Enhancing Your Practice,* I reflected on my path to Reiki. I realized that listening to my intuition played a big part; however, during my actual Reiki I class, taught by Takata-trained Reiki Master Beth Gray, I felt doubts. My mind, honed to a sharply critical voice by my graduate studies, analyzed and dissected everything that my teacher said. By the end of the three-day class, I thought my hands were probably different, but I wasn't sure. Even though I had been guided to learn Reiki, I wasn't prepared to trust Reiki or treat a client anytime soon. The foundation of trust in Reiki that comes from understanding its effectiveness had yet to be established. Eventually, I realized that I would have to go forward at my own pace—practicing on myself, listening to the energy, thinking about the lessons of my experiences, integrating what I had learned, and then listening for guidance once more.

Your path to Reiki is unique, and once you are attuned to Reiki, it's important to move forward at your own pace. There are surprises and wonderful experiences in store for you, but there may also be moments of self-doubt. You must negotiate the path before you one step at a time, going forward only when you feel ready to continue. You can give yourself permission to stay where you are for a while, in order to gain competence and a sense of confidence before moving forward. You can also take "time out" in order to rest or to focus on necessary family or work responsibilities. Your commitment to the journey is not in question. Your patience with the pace of your own progress will allow you to build a foundation of experiences with Reiki that will keep you steady and sure-footed, even if the way becomes difficult or challenging at a later time.

EXPERIENCING "THE FIRST MIRACLE"

"You will have your first miracle," Beth had promised everyone in the Reiki I class—and she was right. A few weeks after that class, I had the opportunity to work on a lame horse, a bay mare named Holly, owned by my best friend, fantasy author Janny Wurts. Since the veterinarian had treated the horse over a period of time without success and finally given up on the case, it was easy to secure Janny's permission to try my hands on Holly's problem hoof. "What have I got to lose?" she asked. We both knew the answer: nothing. She had no expectations or hopes for my success, nor did I.

So we were both surprised and pleased when, soon after I began the Reiki treatment, Holly responded by relaxing, locking her back legs where she stood, and drooping her eyelids—she was drifting off to sleep. This was a relief: my hands would not be trod upon. Meanwhile, as I continued the treatment, I was astonished by the sensations of energy flow that I perceived in my hands: heat, tingling, pulsing, spiraling whorls, even waves that bounced back and forth through Holly's hoof like a well-played Ping-Pong ball. I gaped in amazement. Doing Reiki was actually fun!

Finally, after about forty-five minutes, the energy flow in my hands quieted down. I stood up, dusted off the straw that had stuck to my pants, and promised my friend to return as soon as I was able to repeat the treatment. (My teacher had instructed the class that any chronic condition should be treated with four sessions in a row, like a loading dose of medicine, and then on a regular schedule—once a week or every other week—whatever was convenient to both client and practitioner.)

During the next two weeks, I visited Holly another four times. The day following my last visit, Janny called to tell me that the impossible had happened: Reiki had healed the condition that the veterinarian had been unable to diagnose or treat. Overnight, Holly had extruded three abscesses through the cartilage of the affected hoof, and her lameness had disappeared.

I was astonished and grateful—and intrigued. Surely I, who had no knowledge of horses, had done nothing to help Holly but show up in her barn and extend my hands. Then what—or who—had cured her? My affection and concern for my friend had compelled me to offer to do Reiki. Her trust in me, her open-mindedness to new experiences, and her willingness to allow me to do hands-on healing on her horse had opened the way for a miracle to occur. That miracle healed a horse's lameness, but it also had an impact on my friend and me. After her healing, Holly was sound enough to be ridden again for regular exercise; Janny learned Reiki hands-on healing from Reiki Master Beth Gray at the next Reiki I class Beth taught in our area; and I found myself learning to make room in my understanding of the world for an infinitely healing, absolutely intelligent force that could work through my hands: Reiki, universal life-force energy—Divine Spirit.

TRUSTING THE ENERGY

My gratitude for this first miracle inspired courage. I began to feel comfortable with the thought of offering Reiki to other people. A few weeks later, my friend's writing collaborator, bestselling fantasy author Raymond E. Feist volunteered to be my second client. He had heard about the bay mare's remarkable recovery and now wanted to experience Reiki for himself. He asked if I would treat his congested sinuses. Since I didn't own a bodywork table at the time, I didn't attempt a formal treatment. I positioned a footstool beside one end of a couch, sat in a comfortable position, and floated my hands a few inches above his face. At that point, I didn't *know* that Reiki would work, but based on the success of the treatments on Holly, I was willing to give Reiki a try and hope for the best.

In a very few minutes, Ray asked me if we could take a break so that he could blow his nose. He was sniffling badly. I was terrified. What had I done wrong? I had felt the warmth and tingling radiating from my hands, but had I somehow made his condition worse? My face must have betrayed my concern, because he reassured me.

"This is good," he said, pointing to his red nose. "My sinuses are clearing. The congestion is draining away. I haven't been able to breathe through my nose in six months." He paused to use his handkerchief again. "Now I can breathe," he said and smiled. With that, he tucked the handkerchief into his shirt pocket and lay back down on the couch.

I sighed in relief and sat down again on the footstool to do more Reiki. I decided that I would believe him—and I would trust the energy.

Later, I felt grateful that I had been taught this necessary lesson about the body's natural healing processes by such a kind, direct man who was so appreciative of healing. I felt encouraged by this experience. I *would* go on to offer Reiki to other people. (Of course, I had no idea how central Reiki would become in my life at the time of this treatment, in 1987, or how many people I would go on to treat with Reiki.)

STAYING ON THE PATH

Even after I had experienced success in using Reiki to bring healing to myself and others, I did what many practitioners do: I tested it. If I didn't practice hands-on healing on myself for a day or two, would the energy still be there in my hands, able to bring healing? Or would I lose it through my negligence?

I don't know how many such experiments I conducted in the first year or so of practice, but of course, I discovered that the energy remained with me, no matter how often I put it aside and no matter how far away from spiritual concerns my mind veered. I could give myself a long weekend off from practicing Reiki, and there it would be, as strong as ever, flowing through my hands on Monday morning as I lay in bed with my hands over my heart. At the end of the workday, I could catch an action-thriller movie on TV and feel my mind and emotions reel with the sense of threat, even while the Reiki energy pumped through my hands over my midsection and calmed me.

I loved the fact that there were no "shoulds," no doctrine or dogma or commandments. The very fact that I could choose each day to do Reiki or not was freeing, and I enjoyed that freedom. However, I soon learned that I wanted to experience the relaxation that Reiki brought. I enjoyed that peace of mind. I loved the sensations that I perceived as the energy flowed through my hands; they were fascinating! I felt wonderful when I took the time to do hands-on healing on myself, and I felt humbled and grateful whenever I had the opportunity to offer Reiki to others and witness their healing.

Eventually, I realized that I became cranky and discontented when I didn't do Reiki at least once each day. So I began to do it every day, at least using it to treat myself. Later on, when I learned Reiki distant healing, I began to do Reiki more often, treating myself first thing in the morning as I lay in bed, and in the evening, taking time to send Reiki to others who were in need. Sometimes, however, there were days when I gave myself permission to rush out without doing hands-on healing on myself; I thought, "I have too much to do today. I'm just too busy." I soon discovered that such days didn't seem to go as well and that I didn't enjoy them nearly as much as a day that started out with Reiki.

Little by little, I learned that I love being in the Reiki energy, whether for the duration of a class, the hour or more it may take to do a formal treatment, or the few minutes that it takes to send some distant healing or to do some informal hands-on healing. Not only that, but I love the effects of the Reiki energy on others and myself: it is wonderful and soul satisfying to help someone else feel better, and it is delightful to enjoy a calm mind, a healthy body, and a sense of emotional well-being. For me, these lessons of early practice were accompanied by a gradual transformation in my spiritual awareness: I began to understand that the energy offers the experience of a constant, comforting presence and that its nature is infinitely intelligent, compassionate, and healing.

Do all Reiki practitioners arrive at the same understanding through their practice? Perhaps not, but I think that the energy itself entices us forward on the path of Reiki until we willingly and gladly commit to daily practice. This commitment helps us to heal spiritually. My friends include one Reiki master who was an atheist and another who was an agnostic when they first learned Reiki. They have rethought their worldviews to accommodate the existence of some benevolent higher power or aspect of consciousness that is able to work through them to bring healing. They, too, have made a commitment to daily practice, knowing that it will lead them forward on the path and continue to deepen their understanding of the energy.

JOURNEYING FROM DOUBT TO FAITH TO KNOWLEDGE

In Reiki II class, I ask the students to begin by introducing themselves and sharing a story of some experience with hands-on healing that occurred after they learned Reiki I. In this way, the students are reminded of the issues that they've confronted and their successes with Reiki. Here's a selection of stories from a recent class:

"Soon after I took the Reiki I class, a friend called to invite me to stop by for a visit. As I rang the doorbell and reached for the doorknob, there was this intense surge of Reiki energy in my hands. I couldn't imagine why.

"I heard my friend call out from inside her apartment. She said, 'Come on in, Tina. The door's open.' So I turned the doorknob and pushed the door open into the living room. My friend lay on the couch with a cold compress on her forehead. She told me that she had had a terrible migraine headache all day.

"Now I realized why my hands were so hot! I offered to do some Reiki. She had never heard of it, but she was open to the idea of hands-on healing. I treated her, and her headache went completely away. I was really glad to be able to do that. I was also really surprised that the Reiki energy had started to flow through my hands even before I opened the door, saw her, and realized something was wrong."

The next student in the circle told a story of emotional and mental healing. She said, "Well, nothing like that has ever happened to me, but I did have a good result treating a friend of mine who's a creative artist and a poet. She felt blocked. She couldn't write and was pretty unhappy about it. So I offered to go to her house and give her a Reiki treatment. She had never experienced Reiki before. She said that it made her feel more relaxed than she had felt in a long time. She called me a few days later to tell me that she felt wonderful. She had been able to write and work on a poem the evening after the Reiki treatment. Then, during the week, she had written another nineteen pages for her book. She was really happy."

Everyone was impressed with this success. We smiled and nodded in gratitude, then turned to listen to Lauren Sage, a Reiki master certified in 2005 who asked to assist just so she could be in the energy. "It was 1990 when I learned Reiki I and II from Beth Gray, so it's hard for me to remember one specific experience that happened between the two classes. I do remember that I prayed for guidance about both classes, and it came, too.

"Before the first class, I had to send in fifty dollars as a deposit on the tuition to reserve a space. I thought hard about whether or not to take the class. I wasn't sure what Reiki was and where it came from, and I didn't want to do anything wrong or evil. So I prayed about it each day, whenever I thought about the decision I had to make. I worked as a waitress at the time, and at the end of the week when I gathered up my tips, I had just enough for the deposit. So I sent in a check for fifty dollars with my registration form. That evening, as I swept the restaurant, I found a fifty-dollar bill on the floor. I thought, 'That's a sign! This is something good, and I'm being encouraged to take the class.' My fears went away after that."

She paused to look around the circle. "There was another sign when I learned Reiki II. It was more expensive to take the second-level class, and I thought it would be great to find the money to pay for that class, but it didn't happen that way. Instead, I took the class, and on the way home, as I drove my car, I repeated the name of the third symbol to myself. I wanted to remember it always. I happened to glance out the side window, and I realized that in the passenger seat of the car in the next lane was Beth Gray. One of the assistants at the class was the driver. So as I said the name of the symbol to myself, I looked over at Beth. Then, as I turned my attention back to the road in front of me, I saw a falling star! It was this beautiful trail of light across the night sky, right in the direction I was headed. I understood that as a sign. It confirmed for me what I had experienced, that Reiki is good and that it comes from Spirit. I knew that my path would be guided and lighted."

Such stories are comforting reminders of what all Reiki practitioners eventually come to know. Even though we may have begun our practice of Reiki doubtful of its nature, skeptical of its effectiveness, and uncertain of our own abilities to do hands-on healing, we move through our experiences to a faith in Spirit. This faith is not associated with any particular religion; it is based simply on our trust in Reiki, which is universal, or Spirit-guided, life-force energy. This trust increases day by day, as we stay with the practice of Reiki, experience healing on all levels, and, now and again, witness miracles.

Each of these three stories suggests something more about the nature of Reiki energy than its ability to bring about physical healing. The first story, in which the practitioner described noticing the energy's presence before she was consciously aware of her friend's need for healing, is not unusual, but it does hint that the energy is somehow connected to an all-knowing Source. The second story, in which the practitioner described how her client was healed of a creative block and her creativity was enhanced over the course of the week that followed, suggests that the energy is not only powerfully healing but also life enhancing; it beckons us forward to health, well-being, *and* happiness. The third and final story, presented by a practitioner who prayed and asked for spiritual guidance, shows how prayers can be answered by the energy. Each of these stories was told by a practitioner who was on the way from doubt to trust in the Reiki energy to knowledge of Spirit.

TAKING STEPS TOWARD
A DEEPER UNDERSTANDING

When Reiki students take the advanced course and learn the distant-healing symbols and method, the path of Reiki opens up before them in new ways. The concept of distant, or absent, healing presumes that the power of Reiki transcends geographic distance, and indeed, this is so. How is such healing possible? Reiki, Spirit-guided life-force energy, seems to connect us all and unify us: we are one in Spirit.

However, each of the Reiki symbols focuses the energy in particular ways that reveal even more about the nature and source of the energy.* The first symbol, commonly referred to as the power symbol, calls for an increase in the energy, but it's also profoundly protective. The second symbol, the mental-emotional healing symbol, is calming and tranquilizing, but it also encourages a flow of intuitive impressions between client and practitioner in support of healing that taps the all-knowing aspect of Spirit. The third symbol, the distant-healing symbol, establishes the connection between the practitioner and the absent client so that Reiki healing may occur. The use of the symbol to transcend geographic distances and past, present, and future suggests that Reiki healing occurs in sacred space and time.

Coming to accept the spiritual reality that Reiki distant healing and the symbols imply may take years and many more experiences with Reiki. However, as practitioners we're trained to listen to subtle changes in the energy; we're trained to perceive its flow, its intensity, and its cycles. Eventually, we take time to think about its effectiveness, its source, and the profound sense of blessing that so often accompanies its use in healing. Gently, at our own pace, we move forward into a greater awareness of the spiritual nature of the Reiki energy.

THE FIRST SYMBOL:
POWER AND PROTECTION

A crack of lightning and rumble of thunder made me look up from my desk and out the window of my third-floor home office in a hillside house in the woods. Ominous gray clouds had gathered so low overhead that I wondered if

---

*Traditional practitioners in the Western (Usui Shiki Ryoho) tradition are taught that the symbols are sacred; they are not to be shared with others lightly. As I was taught and continue to teach in this tradition, I will not provide drawings of the symbols for publication, despite my willingness to talk about their use in Reiki practice. Curious readers who are not yet trained as advanced Reiki practitioners can search for drawings of the symbols on the Internet.

they would soon surround the roof. Wind whipped the treetops back and forth in great, sweeping arcs so that they seemed to claw against the sky. How long could they bend like that before one or another of them broke and crashed against the house?

The weather stations had predicted a severe thunderstorm and had issued a tornado advisory. As I watched the roiling clouds grow darker and heard the wind approach a roar, I began to feel frightened and alone. What should I do? What could anyone do against the possible touchdown of a tornado?

Then the answer came to me—not in a lightning flash but after too many to count: I could use the first symbol. As soon as I realized this, I also knew what to do: I moved to the center of the room, stretched out my arms, and visualized the symbol over the house, running vertically down through the roof, through me, through all three floors into the ground, and then spiraling around and around and around, until the energy flowed out my hands in a rush. I chanted the symbol's name. I waited, almost holding my breath, to see what would happen. Within a couple minutes, the winds calmed, the clouds lightened, and a gentle rain began to fall.

I learned later that the tornado did touch down in the antiques district of a town about five miles away. It broke all the display glass in the shops on one side of the street and relocated a couple parked cars, but no one was hurt. Although I'm grateful for the healing focus of the first symbol, that afternoon I felt blessed more than words can tell to know that the energy can focus protection through the first symbol as well.

Like a labyrinth for a walking meditation, the first symbol forces us to focus on what is immediately before us. As we draw its spiral form, we call for the energy to be with us *now* and to be even more strongly present and powerful than in the moment just past. As the spiral narrows, we gather the energy in, so that it's concentrated and focused, and then direct it toward whatever is in need of healing or protection.

If we draw the symbol more than once, it's as if we've repeated a request. We are rewarded with even greater intensification of the energy that flows through our hands. When we use the first symbol in Reiki hands-on healing, repeating it when there's an urgent need, its power is obvious, perceptible to us as increased heat, tingling, and other sensations. However, when we make a habit of drawing or visualizing the first symbol over a steering wheel, on the front door of a house, or on the back of a child setting off for school, even though we aren't doing a Reiki treatment, we're still calling, again and again, for the energy to bring focused healing and protection. While the gesture may feel casual and light-hearted, it offers a quick antidote to worry—and its cumulative effect is extraordinary.

Through the use of the first symbol, we learn that we can ask Spirit for help, healing, and protection, and it will be given to us. "Ask and it shall be given to you," Christ told his apostles, according to the Gospel of Matthew 7:7. When we draw or visualize this symbol, we experience confirmation of Spirit's loving attention to us and abundant provision for our needs.

THE SECOND SYMBOL: MENTAL-EMOTIONAL HEALING AND INTUITIVE INSIGHT

In a Reiki II class in early 2008, I invited the students to practice sending Reiki distant healing back in time. "Does anyone have a specific event or issue from the past that still impacts the present?" I asked.

One practitioner volunteered, "I was in a car accident in April 2005. I still have some physical problems as a result."

"All right, let's all send Reiki distant healing to that event," I suggested. We raised our hands to heart level, named the practitioner as the client, and offered Reiki back in time for her healing on all levels, acknowledging her free will to accept or to reject the offered healing. For the next ten minutes or so, we were all quiet as we sent healing. Then, one by one, we sensed a shift in the energy and concluded the distant-healing session.

After all the practitioners finished taking notes of their impressions, I invited them to share any impressions they received. There was surprising agreement on some of the details of the accident: almost all the practitioners had a visual impression of breaking windshield glass. One described the crushed metal of the vehicle as forming a *c,* with the impact on the passenger side. Most of the practitioners also shared an impression about where the client was most in need of healing: her right leg, lower back, and left shoulder.

Our client nodded in confirmation and admitted the extent of her injuries: "I had a concussion from hitting the windshield. My right leg was broken in two places, and I lost part of my right foot. Some of the ligaments in my shoulder were torn. I was in the hospital for quite a long time."

One of the practitioners asked whether her leg was suspended in the hospital. To this impression, too, she agreed. She went on to describe the bandages and casts she wore.

Finally, I offered my impressions: "I have the sense that the physical injuries are only a part of what you endured. I have the impression that this accident had a much bigger impact on your life than just trauma and time spent in the hospital. The accident wasn't your fault, was it?"

"No," she answered firmly. "It wasn't my fault."

"I sense that when the other car came out of nowhere, it didn't just smash your car and move it over. It derailed your whole life."

She nodded. "It did. I had to stop going to school, and I had to give up my job."

"I had another impression," I told her. "I saw you shooting a gun in a shooting range. It was a black gun, maybe some kind of pistol."

"I did sometimes go to a shooting range back then."

This surprised me. I had thought that the gun might be symbolic.

She continued, "The man I was seeing at the time liked to shoot. I got into it because of him."

Something clicked into place. I told her that there was only one more impression that came to me: "I heard your voice saying, 'I was angry.'"

"I *was* angry. In some ways, I'm still angry."

"He didn't stay with you, did he?" I asked. "The man that you were seeing, he couldn't handle the accident—"

She shook her head no, as if she didn't trust her voice to be steady when she spoke.

"I imagine that you would feel angry about that, too."

"I am," she said, her head high once more.

"It's good that you volunteered to be the client for this practice session.

You can see how Reiki can help you to heal from the effects of the accident on more than just the physical level. It will help you to get your life back on track."

When we use the second symbol in Reiki distant healing to facilitate mental and emotional healing, the energy can bring to light repressed memories and suppressed feelings that the client now needs to consider with conscious awareness in order to claim complete healing. Sometimes, conscious recognition is all that is necessary for healing to occur; at other times, memories and feelings need to be explored and understood in order to be released and forgiven. This is one of the most important uses of intuition in Reiki healing.*

Not every practitioner feels comfortable with the concept of receiving intuitive impressions that may be of value to the client; some also resist the idea of receiving guidance for their own use and direction. However, extending our trust in the energy to guide us in whatever way is for the highest good is a logical next step in the path of Reiki. This step demands both greater trust and a bit of courage: we must admit with complete humility that we do not know in order to be open to knowing; and we must surrender the desire to control the outcome when we agree, on an inner level, to honor the guidance we've received. This step requires faith in the Reiki energy as an expression of Spirit, not as anyone else has defined Spirit but as we have experienced it.

One of the reasons to take this step is to develop a more personal and intimate relationship with Spirit; one of the hallmarks of this relationship is an ongoing "conversation with God," the request for and receiving of inner guidance; one of its blessings is the comforting awareness of a constant, loving Presence that watches over us, gently guides us, and brings us great healing.

---

*For more on this subject and for instruction in specific techniques used in the Western and Japanese traditions, please see my book *Intuitive Reiki for Our Times: Essential Techniques for Enhancing Your Practice.*

THE THIRD SYMBOL: DISTANT HEALING AND CONNECTION TO SPIRIT

Several years ago, as I attuned a Reiki practitioner to the next level, two unusual events occurred: the practitioner coughed throughout the attunement, as if the energy brought up some infection to be healed, and I felt something I had never felt before during an attunement—a comforting sensation of intense warmth around my throat. I didn't interpret the sensation. I attributed it to the energy and let it go. Afterward, the student apologized for coughing so much. She said that she was recovering from strep throat. I encouraged her to go home and rest and do Reiki hands-on healing.

Five days later, at about four o'clock in the afternoon, I felt my throat become very sore. I remembered that I had been exposed to streptococcus bacteria during my student's bout of coughing. Then I recalled the heat that I had felt around my throat during the attunement. I realized that someone must have sent Reiki distant healing back in time to me during those few minutes of exposure, so I set about doing just that. Twenty minutes later, all the pain in

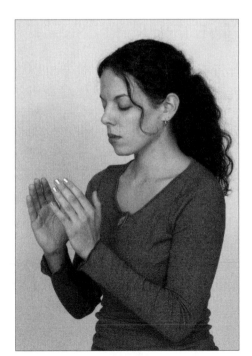

Sending distant healing

my throat had disappeared. Despite my exposure to a highly contagious infection, I remained well.

The third symbol, the distant-healing symbol, is commonly translated from Japanese as a salutation: "God in me greets God in you." This greeting at once acknowledges the Divine within both Reiki practitioner and client, and establishes the location of Reiki healing in sacred time and space. However ordinary the setting for a treatment might seem, it's not ordinary. The Divine is at work and often overcomes any sense of human limitations and accomplishes healing miracles far beyond the expectations and hopes of those providing medical care.

It's for this reason that Reiki distant healing produces such extraordinary results across untold miles. In God, there is no distance. In the energy, there is no distance. Chronological time, too, is shown to be a human construct, unable to limit the energy. In God, past, present, and future are all now. In the energy, all time is now. Sending Reiki healing across time becomes a small matter of expressing human intention, acknowledging free will, and trusting the energy.

THE PATH OF REIKI AND THE PRINCIPLES

When we learn Reiki, we're urged to practice hands-on healing each day on ourselves and offer hands-on healing to others when the opportunity presents itself. By following this recommendation, we can have extraordinary experiences with the energy that teach us that miracles are possible, that we are connected to Spirit, and that our lives aren't as bound by human limitations as we have thought. The energy that flows through our hands, bringing relaxation, peace of mind, and healing, also teaches us about the nature of Spirit, its point of origin. We may learn more about the benevolent, loving, intelligence that is Divine Consciousness than we ever dreamed possible.

Or we may not. We step onto the path of Reiki only when we feel ready to do so, and we proceed at a pace that's comfortable for us. One of the goals we may pursue on this path is to heal ourselves physically, mentally, emotionally, and spiritually so that we may experience wholeness, health, and well-being. For most people, this takes time—years, decades, perhaps a lifetime. It's possible to begin the work of healing and then set it aside to focus more intensely on career or family; five months or five years later, we may decide that, yes, we're ready to resume the work of healing ourselves. Will our hands work? Yes, if we were taught in a traditional way, we were attuned several times, and the channel for Reiki healing is well established. All we need to do is find some quiet place where we won't be interrupted, put our hands in position, and be patient. Eventually—within a half hour or so—the energy will soothe away tension and struggle enough that we are able to notice the sensations in our hands again.

Even those of us who practice Reiki steadily and attain a high level of health and well-being still need to continue to work on self-healing. The commitment to daily self-treatment is a spiritual practice that places us in the flow of the energy; it washes away the negativity that we may have absorbed from our environment or from those around us; it helps us to remain strong and calm in the face of crises; and it bolsters our immune systems, increases longevity, and enhances the overall quality of life. It also reminds us, day after day, that we're connected to Spirit and that our relationship with Spirit can be tender, joyful, and comforting.

The Reiki principles offer us gentle guidelines for returning to the awareness of our connection to Spirit throughout the day, no matter what challenges we face or what blessings come to us. We are granted free will. We may choose to recite the principles morning and night, to be mindful of them throughout the day, or both in order to accelerate our own mental, emotional, and spiritual healing. The principles may become a touchstone for the kind of consciousness we want to experience and express in the world: peaceful, serene, appreciative, honorable, and kind. When we're able to embody these qualities, to live the principles, we demonstrate something of the nature of Spirit that we've come to know through our experiences with Reiki, and we bring healing into our world. This is satisfying to the soul and delightful to the mind. This invites happiness.

SUMMARY

Like Mikao Usui, all Reiki practitioners travel a path to Reiki, and they continue this journey, transformed and still being transformed by the energy, even after they've become practitioners. Many people come to Reiki with significant injuries, illness, or emotional trauma that needs to be healed. They can readily appreciate the importance of daily Reiki self-treatment. Others come to Reiki already having attained health and well-being; they may be eager to use Reiki in service or to further their spiritual development. No matter how we begin, we must accept the conditions of our own beginning and proceed from there to heal, to grow in understanding and wisdom, and to discover how to lead full, happy lives.

The commitment to Reiki practice, including self-treatment, propels us all forward, not only toward greater health and well-being but also to spiritual wholeness and happiness. Why? Reiki is experiential. Whenever we practice on ourselves or others, the energy teaches us something of the nature of Spirit. We're not always conscious that we're learning about peace, compassion, or integrity, but little by little, we absorb this "material"—and integrate the energy of peace, compassion, and integrity into our very being.

The energy also teaches us about the values expressed in the Reiki principles. As we learn how to be patient with ourselves and listen to the energy in our hands, we let go of frustration and anger. As we move from doubt to trust in the energy's effectiveness, we set aside worry. When we witness healing, we feel grateful. The sensitivity of the energy to individual needs and its effectiveness in bringing about complete healing on all levels demonstrates integrity. As we emulate that sensitivity in our relationships with others, we learn to be kind.

The Reiki principles guide us to behave in ways that express the energy. When we meditate on the principles or remember them throughout the day, we remind ourselves to choose peace over anger, and calmness and serenity over worry. We allow ourselves to feel gratitude for all the blessings of our lives. We do our best, and we learn to know ourselves better so that we'll understand what it means to do our best. We look for ways to be kind to others and to ourselves.

Being able to bring healing to others is humbling and awe inspiring, and being able to receive healing is a great blessing. When we attend to the feeling of the energy flowing through our hands each time we practice Reiki, we deepen our understanding of its nature and recognize its origin in Spirit. This connection to Spirit is comforting, tender, and joyful. Practitioners who come to this awareness sometimes realize that in learning Reiki and channeling universal life-force energy through their hands, they've fallen in love with Spirit and with life.

MORE SUGGESTIONS FOR PRACTICE

❧ Reiki accepts us just as we are, and lets us proceed at our own pace. Explore how you came to Reiki, either by writing in a journal or by engaging in deliberate reflection during a walk. Were you experiencing any health problems that prompted you to learn more about Reiki? Are you aware of any emotional baggage from the past that you carried with you? Sometimes, dramatic healing occurs during a Reiki class or in the days that immediately follow. Did you experience such healing? Or are you experiencing healing more gradually, with some improvement in your symptoms each time you practice Reiki on yourself or receive it from another practitioner? Rather than responding to these questions in one sitting, you may want to allow yourself to continue your reflections over several days, at your own pace.

❧ Since learning Reiki hands-on healing, what has healed in your physical body, in your emotional makeup, in your mental attitude, in your spiritual life? Appreciate any and all healing that has occurred. Go into gratitude as if you were entering a church, synagogue, or mosque. Sit in the quietness and be glad for the healing blessings you've received. When you're willing to emerge from this meditation, get out your journal again. Write a thank-you note to all those who were involved in helping you learn about Reiki. This will uplift you even if you never post the note. You may also want to write a thank-you note to the Reiki energy for the healing you've received, or to God if you feel comfortable with that idea. Notice how your physical body responds to the activity of expressing gratitude. Are you smiling? Are you crying tears of joy? The practice of gratitude is also healing.

❧ Go on a walkabout, or just go for a leisurely walk in a beautiful place. As you explore your environment, let yourself explore your inner landscape as well. Think about your pace. Are you walking with a natural stride, swinging your arms at your sides with a sense of ease? Are you racing along and a little out of breath because you're in the habit of rushing everywhere? Or are you strolling, taking lots of time-outs to rest and admire the view? Do you travel the path of Reiki in a similar way? Have you found your stride?

As you walk, also consider the pace of healing that you've experienced since learning Reiki. If you're happy with the results, you may not want to make any changes in your practice, but if you would like to accelerate the pace of healing still more, you may want to commit to daily self-treatment or give more time each day to self-treatment. If you're healthy but want to accelerate your spiritual growth, you may want to look for ways to do Reiki more often for others. Put that thought out to the Universe. Ask Spirit to show you the way.

❧ Exploring the inner landscape of the mind and heart is very much like walking the land: you can find pleasure in moving forward at a gentle pace and observing the beauty around you, but troublesome issues can also rise to the surface of conscious awareness and block the way. The Reiki principles can help us resolve such issues so that we can move forward again; they also offer a peaceful way of being in the world that calls forth our innate good. Think about how much importance you've given to the Reiki principles in your life as a practitioner so far. If you would like to improve your understanding of their value, you'll need to integrate them into your consciousness.

There are many ways to do this. You might try meditating on them twice a day, reciting them morning and night, as Mikao Usui recommended. You might write them down on several pieces of sticky-backed paper and place them wherever you'll be likely to see them throughout the day: on a mirror, the dashboard of your car, the wall of your office cubicle, and so on. Then read them repeatedly, as if they were affirmations. You might also focus on each of the Reiki principles in turn, beginning with "just for today, do not anger," and allow yourself to be guided by the principle in your behavior until you feel you've mastered it. Then go on to the next. There's no one right way to become more mindful of the Reiki principles. The path of Reiki is a gentle one. Enjoy the ability to proceed at your own pace. Claim the Reiki principles as tools for personal transformation and peace in your own time.

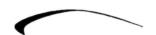

2

THE REIKI PRINCIPLES

In March 1987, in my level I class, when I first heard of the Reiki principles, I was more preoccupied with learning how to do Reiki hands-on healing than I was with remembering the details of the many stories told by my teacher, Takata-trained Reiki Master Beth Gray. Although I listened attentively on the final day of class as Beth mentioned the Reiki principles during the conclusion of the story of Mikao Usui's life and his meditation on Mt. Kurama, I let them go. Surely these simple statements were written down somewhere! I could look them up later. There was so much else that Beth had said—and was still saying—that seemed more important to remember: how Reiki healing works on all levels—physical, mental, emotional, and spiritual; how to use Reiki healing as complementary medicine; how to place the hands for self-treatment and for client treatment.

Two days before, when Beth had first said to the class, "Listen to your hands!" and described the many sensations we might experience as we performed Reiki, I had given her my complete attention. Now, after many hours of instruction, questions and answers, and practice, I believed I understood clearly how to give a Reiki treatment; I thought I knew how to recognize the healing flow and how to register the subtle changes that would signal that it was time to move to the next position. Understanding how to use my hands to do Reiki felt so completely urgent that I listened to my teacher as if the knowledge she imparted might save someone's life—maybe even my own.

And, of course, it has. Like many Reiki practitioners and teachers, I've watched Reiki change a prognosis from poor to positive; I've heard doctors with beaming smiles say, "We don't know why, but . . ."; and I've sat at the bedsides of ill and injured people and offered them Reiki's pain relief, accelerated healing, and comforting touch. So perhaps I was right to attend so closely to my teacher's every word about the Reiki energy and how to offer Reiki treatment. Many Reiki practitioners still make the same choice.

A few weeks after the class, perhaps because I did listen so closely and selectively, I was able to introduce a new acquaintance to Reiki as a form of hands-on healing by demonstrating the hand positions and describing the sensations he could expect to feel during treatment. He was receptive—and so delighted with the results that he soon learned Reiki himself. However, if he had asked me about the Reiki principles, I think I would have made some excuse to him. They had seemed so much less important to me than learning Reiki itself during the class that I probably would have had to check my notes and call him back!

A few years after learning Reiki, while assisting at one of Beth's classes, I received one of her new business cards, double folded on pale, blue-gray stock. On the front of the card, there was a beautiful photo portrait of Beth, smiling and radiant, positioned above her name, "Rev. Beth Gray." Inside the card, on the upper panel, were her business address and contact information; on the lower panel was a brief list of her professional qualifications, beginning with "Reiki Master Teacher and Practitioner." These two panels were spanned by a line drawing of a single rose, a symbol of love, beauty, and perfection that Beth had adopted to convey the experience of Reiki. Finally, on the back panel, printed in the same bold type, she presented the Reiki principles:

REIKI IDEALS

Just for today—
Do not worry, Accept
Do not anger, Accept

Count your blessings
Do an honest day's work
Be kind to all living things

This was a lovely, gentle way to demonstrate to her students the value she placed on the Reiki principles and to communicate to all her professional contacts that she lived by spiritual precepts that promoted peace, compassion, and kindness.

She had another way to help us appreciate the Reiki principles that was also simple and effective but so subtle that I didn't even know it was happening until after I had assisted at several Reiki I classes and realized that she usually presented her class material in the same sequence. Just before each of the four attunements she gave to students in a level I class, she would tell part of the story of Mikao Usui's life and vision on Mt. Kurama. Then, after each of the four attunements, as students experienced the energy flowing into them and transforming them, Beth led everyone in meditation. The first of these meditations focused on letting go of worry, anger, and fear. "Just for today," she urged us, "accept." The second of the meditations recommended that we learn to appreciate our lives with heartfelt gratitude. The third encouraged us always to "do an honest day's work" and strive to do our best. The last of the meditations celebrated the power of kindness.

Often students who still felt the powerful effects of attunement to the Reiki energy found themselves quietly moved to tears, releasing and healing past grievances, and opening up to hope and the possibility of happiness. Beth led all of these meditations against a background of softly played music that she had chosen, an instrumental piece called "Prelude to Lazaris," channeled by Lazaris (Jack Purcell). This musical work conveys the overcoming of melancholy through hope, effort, and inspiration, culminating in the triumphant exaltation of the human spirit. It was, indeed, a perfect tonal accompaniment to the meditations.

Each of the meditations lasted perhaps a half hour, although Beth's soothing, hypnotic voice made it easy to lose all track of time. Because Beth taught these Reiki I classes over a long weekend (Friday evening, all day Saturday, and Sunday afternoon), she was able to do one attunement and meditation on the first day of class, two attunements and meditations on the second day, and one attunement and meditation on the final day, when she would also complete the story of Mikao Usui.

So how was it that I left my own Reiki I class with so little grasp of the importance of the Reiki principles? Perhaps it was because I listened to these guided meditations with "half an ear," giving them only a fraction of my attention as I focused on the energetic aftereffects of each attunement. Or perhaps because I heard Beth say that Reiki is not a religion, that it has no doctrine or dogma, I relegated the principles to "interesting historical background" and promptly forgot them. Certainly, I regarded them as nonessential to the practice of hands-on healing.

And so they are. It's absolutely possible to learn Reiki, to be properly attuned to the energy, and to practice on oneself and others without giving the principles more than a passing thought. Yet because Reiki masters who teach in a traditional way are required to provide a history of Reiki during their level I classes, almost all new Reiki practitioners receive at least a brief introduction to the Reiki principles; how much importance they're given is up to the teacher.

THE TRANSLATOR'S WORK

If you look up the word *translation* in a dictionary, you'll see that it means more than to study a text, analyze its meaning, and then compose a text that conveys the same meaning in another language. While this is the task that a translator faces, it's never easy. In all languages, words may have one or more denotations (the meaning or set of meanings found in a dictionary); most words also have connotations (subtle associations or shades of meaning that have become associated with the word through its use in spoken and written language within a lively, dynamic culture). Adding to this complexity, many words have a long, rich history of associations that have accrued to them over centuries of use.

To obtain a rough translation, a translator might attempt to replace each word in a primary text with a word with the same denotations in another language. However, the diversity of cultures and environments around the world makes a one-to-one correspondence between words across languages impossible. For example, how would a translator convey the word *sandstorm* in the Inuit language or the word *frostbite* in the Bedouin language?

To make the task even more daunting, characters in some languages, including Japanese and Chinese, are ideographic or pictographic; that is, the "letter" is drawn in such a way that it communicates part of the meaning of the whole word. Within the Japanese language, the characters called *kanji* are particularly rich in meaning, because they've been used in communication between Japan and China for centuries. The word *Reiki* itself is composed of two kanji, some of the Reiki symbols are composed of kanji, and the Reiki principles are also composed of kanji.

To accurately translate the Reiki principles from Japanese into any other language is a worthy undertaking and a challenging task. We're fortunate to have translations into English from the original by Frank Arjava Petter and Chetna Kobayashi, Hiroshi Doi, Hyakuten Inamoto, and others. These translations alone, with their slight differences in placement and emphasis, might provoke some discussion and invite further study. However, we also have Hawayo Takata's presentation of the Reiki principles to consider, as remembered by her students. The variety of ways in which Takata rendered the principles into English suggests that she had a sense of the richness of their original meaning in Japanese, even if she was unaware of the Japanese titles given to the principles by Mikao Usui or his recommendation to recite the principles twice a day. In any case, thinking about both the direct translations and the many paraphrases of the translations is a way to arrive at a deeper understanding and appreciation of the Reiki principles and their place in Reiki practice.

TRADITIONAL PRESENTATION
OF THE REIKI PRINCIPLES IN THE WEST

Reiki practitioners who learned Reiki from one of the twenty-two Reiki masters initiated by Hawayo Takata between 1976 and 1980 have usually been presented with the Reiki principles in the context of the long story Takata told of Mikao Usui's life: After being transformed by the Reiki energy that came to him at the end of his twenty-one-day meditation on Mt. Kurama, Mikao Usui returned to the temple where he had lived as a monk for some time to consult the abbot about how he should offer Reiki healing to the world. After additional meditation, fasting, and prayer, he and the abbot decided that he should begin his service in the Beggar City, a poor, crime-ridden section of Kyoto where there were many sick and lame people. Usui worked for years, treating the beggars for free, until one beggar's lack of appreciation for the blessing of Reiki caused him to reflect on the importance of gratitude. He left the Beggar City never to return and realized the importance of the values expressed in the Reiki principles.

Yet even though the story of Mikao Usui's life, as Takata taught it, was faithfully passed along by the Reiki masters she initiated, there were some differences in how they presented the Reiki principles and how they remembered Takata's presentation of them. Consider the following examples:

Before her death in 1980, Hawayo Takata asked Helen J. Haberly, one of her Reiki students, to write the story of her life. The book that resulted, *Reiki: Hawayo Takata's Story,* tells of many of the most important events in Takata's life, and it also summarizes her story of the origins of Reiki, including Mikao Usui's encounter with the beggars.

> He [Mikao Usui] realized that although he had been very successful in balancing the physical bodies of the beggars, he had had no concern for their spiritual health. At this time he added to Reiki his Five Spiritual Precepts:
>
> > *Just for today, do not worry.*
> > *Just for today, do not anger.*
> > *Honor your neighbors, your parents, your friends.*
> > *Give thanks for all living things.*
> > *Earn your living honestly.*[1]

Notice that the third Reiki principle, the practice of gratitude, is no longer the central principle but is assigned to fourth place. A recommendation to "honor" friends and family is now in the third position. What most Reiki practitioners would recognize as the fifth Reiki principle, the encouragement to practice kindness, is not present.

In her book *Living Reiki: Takata's Teachings,* Fran Brown, one of the original twenty-two Reiki masters trained by Hawayo Takata, offers this account of the same episode in Usui's life, as told by Takata:

> He refused to treat beggars because of their lack of gratitude.
> He returned to the monastery and talked with the old monk.
> Then he devised the following creed to be taught along with counseling and the cause of the ailment.

> > *Just for today: Do not ANGER*
> > *Just for today: Do not WORRY*
> > *Just for today: COUNT YOUR BLESSINGS, honor*
> > > *your parents, teachers, and neighbors. Eat food with*
> > > *gratitude*
> > *Just for today: LIVE HONESTLY*
> > *Just for today: BE KIND TO ALL LIVING THINGS*[2]

In this version of the Reiki principles, the first and second principles have changed places. In third place, there is now a long admonition to practice gratitude *and* the honoring of ancestors and other "elders." Note that Mikao Usui is now credited with the writing, "the devising," of the Reiki principles as well.

Another source, *Early Days of Reiki: Memories of Hawayo Takata*, compiled by Anneli Twan, daughter of Takata-trained Reiki Master Wanja Twan, offers this version of the Reiki principles from the class notes of Mary Hodwitz, who learned Reiki I from Takata in June 1979 and Reiki II from Takata in October 1979:

> These are the Reiki ideals as Takata taught them . . .

> > *Just for today, not to anger.*
> > *Just for today, not to worry.*
> > *Count your blessings, give thanks for food, for water, for*
> > > *parents, for friends, for fresh air.*
> > *Earn your living honestly.*
> > *Be kind to everything that has life.*[3]

Notice that once again, the third Reiki principle, practice gratitude, has changed and become more inclusive: we are to practice gratitude for everything in nature and for everyone who nurtures us, from our family of origin to our friends.

Did Hawayo Takata present the Reiki principles in a consistent way or not? Certainly, the sense of them remains intact across these three sources, although some details of presentation do not agree. If these are actual quotations from Takata, it seems possible that some of Takata's comments on the meaning have become incorporated into the principles themselves. Another possibility is that these are not quotations but paraphrases of Takata from memory, which would necessarily be less precise.

This method of presenting the Reiki principles, within the context of Takata's story of Mikao Usui's life and vision, was preserved through the 1980s and most of the 1990s by the Reiki masters she taught who traveled worldwide, and by later generations of Reiki masters teaching in the same tradition. In fact, some traditional Reiki masters continue to teach the Reiki principles in the context of Takata's story today, despite the challenges to the accuracy of its details that arose in the late 1990s.

THE TRADITIONAL JAPANESE PRESENTATION OF THE PRINCIPLES

On the eve of the millennium, the winds of change blew around the world, bringing wonderful news from Japan: not only was there an organization of Reiki practitioners and teachers in Japan (Usui Reiki Ryoho Gakkai) that had been founded during Mikao Usui's time, but it still existed; its members still met monthly; and it had its own tradition of Reiki techniques and attunements, and its own version of Reiki history and the Reiki principles. Of course, this news did not reach the rest of the world all at once, nor was it easily accepted by all who heard it.

In 1997, a photo of Mikao Usui, with a more complete version of the principles written in Japanese calligraphy above his image, appeared in a book called *Reiki Fire: New Information about the Origins of the Reiki Power—A Complete Manual,* by Frank Arjava Petter.[4] Along with this image, Petter offered a surprising translation of the memorial to Usui that marks his grave outside Saihoji Temple in Tokyo. The author of the long inscription on the stone marker, which stands several feet tall, is Navy Rear Admiral Juzaburo Gyuda, the first chairperson of the Gakkai to succeed Mikao Usui.[5] This inscription provides many details of Mikao Usui's life, his ancestry, and his accomplishments. It describes the long meditation and fast on Mt. Kurama that culminated in his enlightenment and empowerment to do Reiki healing, and chronicles his career as a spiritual teacher and healer who touched the lives of thousands of people throughout Japan during his lifetime. Mikao Usui's legacy, the inscription proclaims, may bring hope for healing to the whole world.

Within the text is an encouragement to practice Reiki and meditate upon the Reiki principles.

Reiki not only heals diseases, but also amplifies innate abilities, balances the spirit, makes the body healthy, and thus helps achieve happiness. To teach this to others you should follow the five principles of the Meiji Emperor and contemplate them in your heart.

They should be spoken daily, once in the morning and once in the evening.

> *1. Don't get angry today.*
> *2. Don't worry today.*
> *3. Be grateful today.*
> *4. Work hard today (meditative practice).*
> *5. Be kind to others today.*

The ultimate goal is to understand the ancient secret method for gaining happiness (Reiki) and thereby discover the all-purpose cure for many ailments. If these principles are followed, you will achieve the great tranquil mind of the ancient sages.[6]

How did this translation become available? Petter, a German-born Reiki master who had lived in Japan for several years, and his Japanese wife, Chetna M. Kobayashi, had made a sincere effort to discover more about the early history of Reiki. One of their own Reiki students, Ms. Shizuko Akimoto, knew of their interest and their attempts to research this subject. When an older gentleman named Mr. Tsutomu Oishi began visiting Ms. Akimoto for treatments and casually mentioned that "'. . . there is a natural healing technique called

Reiki,'"[7] she felt hopeful that he might know more of how Reiki had originally been taught in Japan.

Over the course of several conversations, Mr. Oishi explained to Ms. Akimoto that he himself had learned Reiki sometime in the 1950s. He also showed her the photograph of Mikao Usui that had been passed down to him.[8] Ms. Akimoto recognized that the photo provided important evidence of Usui's life and work in teaching Reiki throughout Japan, and she contacted Reiki Master Frank Petter to tell him about Mr. Oishi and his story. Petter did some further research, which led him to visit Saihoji Temple, where the Usui Memorial is located, and to undertake the translation of the inscription; then he organized the new information and some of his own teaching materials into manuscript form. The volume that resulted, *Reiki Fire,* was published in both German and English, and immediately began to open the minds of Reiki practitioners and teachers worldwide to a new view of Reiki history.

Still, Frank Arjava Petter continued his research and translation work. During the year that followed publication of *Reiki Fire,* he turned his attention to the more complete text of the Reiki principles that Mr. Oishi had also made available to him. Petter offered his translation in *Reiki: The Legacy of Dr. Usui:*

THE SECRET METHOD OF INVITING HAPPINESS
THE WONDERFUL MEDICINE FOR ALL DISEASES
(OF THE BODY AND THE SOUL)

> *Just today*
> *1. Don't get angry*
> *2. Don't worry*
> *3. Show appreciation*
> *4. Work hard (on yourself)*
> *5. Be kind to others*

Mornings and evenings, sit in the gassho position . . . and repeat these words out loud and in your heart.
[For the] improvement of body and soul, Usui Reiki Ryoho.

THE FOUNDER, MIKAO USUI[9]

What's remarkable about this translation is that it gives us a new double-title for the Reiki principles that offers the promise of both happiness and health to those who practice Reiki. The instruction to say the principles twice daily, signed by "the founder, Mikao Usui," is also new. Note that the fourth principle, which Petter had previously presented in *Reiki Fire* as "Work hard today (meditative practice)," he now translates as "Work hard (on yourself)."

Meanwhile, in Japan, another important event had occurred: in May 1998, the first Japanese book about Reiki, *Iyashino Gendai Reiki-ho: Modern Reiki Method for Healing,* was published. When news of the book's publication reached the West, Canadian, American, and British Reiki masters decided to invite the book's author, Mr. Hiroshi Doi, to visit the West.[10] To their surprise, he promptly accepted. In August 1999, in Vancouver, British Columbia, Mr. Doi conducted a three-day workshop on Reiki's early history and traditional and modern Reiki methods, before an enthusiastic and interested audience of Reiki masters who had gathered together from all over the world. He did so with the knowledge and permission of the Gakkai, of which he is a member, and shared information with a generosity of spirit that brought great healing to all those who attended.

The workshop was so successful that the sponsors decided to invite Mr. Doi to repeat it the following year, and he kindly agreed. During that year, *Iyashino Gendai Reiki-ho* was successfully translated into English, and the workshop was expanded to international conference size. It was repeated annually through 2004, by which date Mr. Doi was traveling worldwide to teach traditional Usui Reiki Ryoho and Gendai Reiki.

The English translation of *Iyashino Gendai Reiki-ho* by Akiko Kawarei and others, which Mr. Doi approved, included another new and more complete translation of the Reiki principles:

SECRET METHOD TO INVITE HAPPINESS
MIRACLE MEDICINE FOR ALL DISEASES

> *Just for today, do not get angry.*
> *Do not be grievous.*
> *Express your thanks.*
> *Be diligent in your business, and be kind [to] others.*

Gassho and repeat them in mind at the beginning and the end of each day.
Usui Reiki Ryoho—Improve your mind and body

FOUNDER
MIKAO USUI[11]

The Reiki principles, which Mr. Doi calls "the Five Admonitions," are to be regarded as a "guide to a way of life . . ."[12] His translation is based on a copy of the Japanese calligraphy in Mikao Usui's own handwriting, given to him by Ms. Kimiko Koyama, one of his teachers and the most recent past chairperson of the Gakkai.

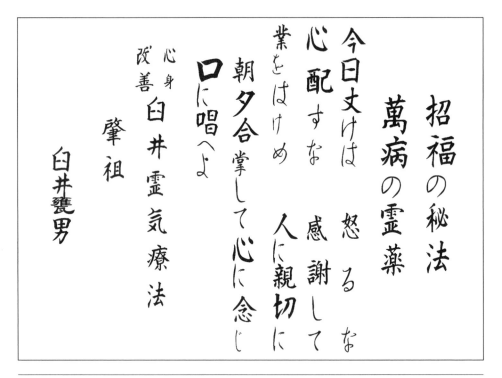

The Gainen, the Reiki principles in their complete form, are read from top to bottom and right to left. The titles are in the two columns at far right, followed by the familiar core concepts (in the third to fifth columns from the right). The recommendation to perform gassho and recall the principles throughout the day are next (in the sixth and seventh columns). Then Mikao Usui identifies his system (the eighth column), his role as founder of the system (the ninth column), and his name (the tenth and final column) at the far left.

THE ORIGINAL AUTHOR OF
THE REIKI PRINCIPLES

Some of the Reiki masters trained by Hawayo Takata understood that the Reiki principles, adopted by Mikao Usui as spiritual precepts, were written by the Meiji Emperor; others thought that Mikao Usui was the author of the principles. Without a source document at hand, there was apparently some confusion and no easy way to resolve that confusion for students.

Frank Arjava Petter, in *Reiki Fire,* and Hiroshi Doi, in *Iyashino Gendai Reiki-ho,* credit the Meiji Emperor as the author of the Reiki principles. Bronwen and Frans Stiene, in *The Reiki Sourcebook,* present two translations of the Meiji Emperor's "Imperial Rescript on Education," which would have been available to Mikao Usui and might have offered a conceptual source.[13] After the publication of his book, however, Mr. Doi made an interesting discovery while browsing in a Japanese bookshop that raised the possibility that the original author was someone else: Dr. Suzuki Bizan, author of *Kenzen-no-genri,* a book published in 1914. The title of Bizan's book can be translated as "A Path to Soundness."[14]

Mr. Doi shared this rather startling news at the September 2002 Usui Reiki Ryoho Conference in Toronto, Canada. His friend and colleague, Reiki Master Hyakuten Inamoto, provides more details about this discovery in *Komyo Reiki Kai: Reiki Healing Art,* the teaching manual he created for Komyo Reiki, his synthesis of traditional Japanese and Western Reiki techniques. He writes: "the phrase titled 'A Path to Soundness' reads: 'Today only / Be not angry, / Be not fearful, / With honesty, / Perform diligently your duty, / Be kind to others. / By Bizan."[15]

Who was Dr. Suzuki Bizan? What was his contribution to Japanese culture when he wrote this book? What was the content of his book? Was Dr. Bizan a doctor of medicine or a scholar, or was he, like Mikao Usui, given the title of "doctor" to honor the healing work he performed? Did he and Usui ever meet in person? How did Usui come across his book? What impact did reading this book have on Usui's thoughts and way of life? Did he read it in 1914, when it was first published, or at some later time? Did he read the whole book because he found it helpful in its entirety, or was he inspired only by those few lines on the opening page of "A Path to Soundness" that became the Reiki principles?

What idea or impulse prompted Mikao Usui to adopt this brief passage as a useful source for spiritual guidance for his students? Did he regard the precepts as sufficient for the attainment of "soundness" or wholeness? If so, why did he leave off the original title in recopying the principles for his students' use and replace it with a double title of his own making: "The Secret Method of Inviting Happiness/The Miracle Medicine for All Diseases"? If Reiki healing offers "the miracle medicine for all diseases," does the practice of these five spiritual precepts bring happiness? Can he possibly mean that Reiki healing invites happiness into our hearts as well? Or is it possible that the practice of the five precepts alone is sufficient to bring us both happiness and health?

These titles are enticing. They invite us to practice Reiki—and to reflect on the Reiki principles—with a sense of unlimited possibility: the Reiki way of healing mind and body leads to happiness and miracles. The puzzle we are left to work out is one of measure and proportion. When so much of our practice offers us the opportunity to directly experience the Reiki energy as we do hands-on and distant healing, and this experience by itself is healing and transforming, what part do the Reiki principles have in our lives? Can twice-daily recitation of the principles in some way support our happiness or accelerate our healing? Can it open us to deeper, richer experiences of the energy as we do treatments on others or on ourselves? For every Reiki practitioner, there's a simple way to find out: follow Mikao Usui's recommendation. Recite the principles twice daily. Be mindful of them in everyday life.

There's a third view of the origins of Reiki that deserves to be carefully considered, even though it's much less well known and doesn't accord with either the account of Usui's life inscribed on the memorial stone outside Saihoji Temple or with Hawayo Takata's story about the turning point in Usui's life: his twenty-one-day fast and meditation on Mt. Kurama, which ended with his transformation into a spiritual teacher and healer. In *O-Sensei: A View of Mikao Usui,* Dave King shares a perspective on Usui's teachings that he learned from Tenon-in, a Buddhist nun who was associated with Usui from 1920 until his death in 1926.[16] She herself died at the age of 107 in 2005. King's research on Usui-do, the Usui system of mind and body healing, began in 1971, when he studied with Yuki Onuki, a teacher of the Usui method initiated by Toshihiro Eguchi, one of Usui's closest disciples. In addition, King studied with Tatsumisan, who learned the Usui method from Chujiro Hayashi between 1927 and 1931, about five years before Hawayo Takata traveled to Japan and became a patient and then a student of Hayashi.

Although much is remarkable about the view of Usui's life and work presented in *O-Sensei: A View of Mikao Usui,* the element of most interest for the purpose of this book is the importance placed on the Reiki principles. King writes that, like a teacher of a martial art, Mikao Usui had a dojo or training hall with a dozen mats for meditation and other exercises. On entering the dojo, a student would bow to Usui and then in the direction of the *tokonoma,* an alcove in the wall opposite the entry, which contained a hanging scroll. In Usui's dojo, the writing on the scroll was of the Gainen—the text of the original Reiki principles—in its complete form, including the two titles, the Gokai (which we refer to as the five principles or ideals), and the signature. According to Tenon-in, Mikao Usui took brush in hand "to write a set of simple concepts that were to form the basis of this system" in early 1921.[17] Toshihiro Eguchi became a member of Usui's dojo the same year and introduced a palm healing method in 1923 that "expanded on Usui's ideas and made use of prayer and other religious practices."[18] This sets Usui and his followers on the spiritual path that culminates in Reiki, as we know it today, at approximately the same time that his spiritual transformation on Mt. Kurama is believed to have occurred by the Gakkai, and it establishes these simple precepts for harmony in mind and body as key to his own practice and that of his earliest students.

Through the work of Frank Arjava Petter, Hiroshi Doi, Hyakuten Inamoto, Dave King, and many others, we now know much more about the early history of Reiki in Japan. Its origins appear to be complex and may never be fully known and understood, or even well documented. Many of the parable-like episodes in Takata's story of Mikao Usui's life have been discounted as embellishments of the tale for the pleasure of a Western, and primarily Christian, audience. Yet she featured Mikao Usui's meditation and vision on Mt. Kurama as the spiritual turning point in his life, just as it is recorded on the memorial stone that marks his grave and as is taught by the Gakkai; and she encouraged her students to embrace the Reiki principles, just as the author of the memorial stone inscription does. Yet it's not the moment on Mt. Kurama that Tenon-in described to Dave King but the spiritual discipline of the dojo, the reverence for the Gainen, and the living of the Reiki principles, which she believed to be the central spiritual teaching of Mikao Usui.

NOW YOU: LEARN MORE ABOUT REIKI'S BEGINNINGS

Take the time to learn more about the origins of Reiki and the Reiki principles. It's possible not only to read Frank Petter's and Hiroshi Doi's books but also to study with them, for both travel around the world teaching Reiki. Dave King now lives in China but occasionally travels to teach in other countries. Read *O-Sensei: A View of Mikao Usui* for another perspective on Usui's life and spiritual practice and contact King through the website http://threshold.ca/usui-do for more information about his classes. If you would rather be an armchair traveler, visit www.threshold.ca, which offers detailed information on early Reiki history and practice within the Gakkai. The site includes the Japanese text of the Reiki principles from the Reiki Ryoho Hikkei, the manual used by Mikao Usui for his students, and yet another interesting translation.

PRINCIPLES, PRECEPTS, OR IDEALS?

Because Hawayo Takata, the first Westerner to learn Reiki and teach it widely, presented these five statements as the Reiki principles or the Reiki ideals, they're best known throughout the world by this brief title. With recent and more complete translations from the original Japanese text now available, we know that Mikao Usui gave his own double title to these guidelines for living: "The Secret Method of Inviting Happiness/The Miracle Medicine for all Diseases." Although his titles are far more suggestive of the power and promise of Reiki as spiritual pathwork, their wordiness makes it unlikely that they'll come into common use. In books and online, it's likely that Reiki masters worldwide will continue posting "The Reiki Principles" for their students and others interested in learning more about Reiki.

However, if we choose to use such abbreviated titles as "The Reiki Principles," we must remain aware of the danger that the purpose of the principles may be misunderstood; and this has to do with denotative meaning.

Principles can mean "moral guidelines," or it can mean "rules." The word *precepts* can also mean "rules," but it also carries with it the sense of "aspirations" or "ideals." The word *ideals,* which Takata also used, suggests that these are statements of what we hope to realize or achieve, although we may never fully succeed. In practicing and in teaching Reiki, it's worthwhile to give this issue some thought. What title would you choose to honor the Reiki tradition in which you were taught and to communicate that these words are encouragement to live a happy, healthy life of spiritual worth?

"JUST FOR TODAY"

This brief phrase appears in all the direct translations and almost all paraphrases of translations. The simple words, "just for today," invite us to be gentle with ourselves in attempting to live by the Reiki principles. These words center us in the present moment. Whatever our faults, whatever our past wrongs, we are encouraged to set aside our sense of failure and begin to be who we truly are, at our best—now. Whatever difficulties we face, however overwhelmed we may feel, we're urged to set aside all worry for the moment. Let us appreciate all that is good in our lives now. Whatever our hopes and ambitions, let's do the best we can today. With heartfelt gratitude for the good in our lives and with self-respect and integrity, surely we can be kind to everyone we encounter today—including the person we see in the mirror.

The phrase "just for today" helps us to narrow our focus to the present moment and our attention to the creation of good. We can use this phrase to remind ourselves that we're not limited by the past, nor are we necessarily freed of all limitations in the future. We are what we are—right now. We can best address whatever challenges we face by being willing to be present, to be fully conscious of all the facts, aware of all the feelings. When we're willing to be fully present to each moment of our experience and do our best, each day offers us many satisfactions, many achievements, many simple pleasures and delights.

However much we might enjoy reminiscing about the past or daydreaming about the future, now is the moment when we're most fully conscious. It's up to us to practice peace, serenity, gratitude, integrity, and kindness "just for today" in order to discover what difference such a day makes. Do we find that we've made a friend of an enemy? Does a solution to a problem come to mind? Does joy awaken in us out of appreciation for the blessings in our lives? Do we feel better about who we are because we've done the best we can? Do we feel a sense of kinship with a stranger because we've made the effort to be kind? When we practice the Reiki principles "just for today," the impact of that choice in the moment ripples out like a wave across the surface of water, changing the quality of our interactions with everyone and our experience of ourselves for hours or even days afterward. Practicing the Reiki principles moment by moment changes us and heals us, improving the quality of our lives.

THE VALUE OF THE REIKI PRINCIPLES

Just as in Japan, Reiki practitioners and teachers trained worldwide in the Western tradition are encouraged to understand the value that Mikao Usui placed on the Reiki principles. However, because Hawayo Takata presented Mikao Usui's adoption of the Reiki principles as a result of his encounter with the ungrateful beggar—a single incident in the much longer story she told of his life—most practitioners see this as his personal choice: he turns away from the beggar's foolishness and instead turns toward wisdom, intent on embracing the healthy, spiritual values expressed by the Reiki principles. Here is a retelling of the episode:*

When Mikao Usui descended from Mt. Kurama, transformed and healed by the experience of Reiki energy after his long meditation, fast, and prayer vigil, he knew that Reiki healing was to be his work, but he did not know where to begin. He consulted with the abbot of the order at the temple where he had found the scroll. After another day and night of meditation, fasting, and prayer, he and the abbot decided that he should begin to offer healing to the sick and the lame in the Beggar City, that part of Kyoto where the Beggar King ruled. Here, there was a very great need for healing.

So it was that for the next few years, Usui dedicated his life to treating the beggars. Many came to him seeking healing from leprosy, tuberculosis, and

---

*For a retelling of the complete story, see *Traditional Reiki for Our Times*, pages 75–84.

other diseases. Always, he encouraged those who were cured to appreciate the great blessing of healing that they had received and to make the most of the rest of their lives. He urged them to go to the center of Kyoto to find work and a place to live. Some of them, he hoped, might even marry, have families, and in all ways, enjoy the full happiness of life.

Then one day, a beggar who seemed strangely familiar came to Mikao Usui requesting treatment.

"Don't I know you?" Mikao Usui asked, studying the man's face.

"Oh yes, Dr. Usui," the beggar replied. "I have been here before, some years ago."

"Didn't I treat you with Reiki until you were well?"

"Yes, Dr. Usui. You treated me until I was completely cured."

"Then why are you here again for treatment? Didn't you leave the Beggar City to find work?"

"Yes, I did, Dr. Usui. I found work and a place to live, just as you advised. I worked very hard all day. At night, I came home, and even though I was very tired, I cooked a little rice and vegetables to eat. Then after dinner, I fell asleep. And the next day, I woke again at dawn and did the same, again and again and again, day after day after day. After a long time of working so hard, I decided that it was much easier to be a beggar. So I returned to the Beggar City and took up my old profession. I have been out begging in the cold and the wind and the rain, and now I am sick."

Mikao Usui was not given to anger, but he was upset by this man's confession of laziness and by his ingratitude for the healing he had already received. So Usui did not treat the beggar. Instead, he turned on his heel and walked away, straight out of the Beggar City. Never again, he decided, would he give away Reiki to someone who did not appreciate its value. He walked into the business district of Kyoto, found a torch, lit it, and held it high, even though it was the middle of the day. Then he called out to passersby that he could offer healing treatments. Many people came to him, happy to pay a small amount to receive the priceless gift of health and well-being.

And, as a result of this encounter with the beggar, Mikao Usui adopted the five Reiki principles: Just for today, do not anger and do not worry. Be grateful. Do an honest day's work. Be kind.

How could the Reiki principles have become so important to Usui as a result of this single incident? Rather than becoming angry with the ungrateful beggar, Usui chose to walk away from the conflict, indicating that he would not allow the beggar or anyone else to devalue the worth of his healing work or of Reiki. He decided instead to leave the Beggar City, to go away from a familiar place, an established routine, and a known source of support to venture into the "unknown territory" of downtown Kyoto to declare that he was open for business. Would anyone be willing to come to him to pay for the Reiki healing treatment that he offered? Just for that day, he did not worry.

The intense emotion that he felt was transmuted into constructive action: he made the decision to go forth from the Beggar City to seek out clients who would pay him as a token of their appreciation for his time and energy and as an indication of their gratitude for the quality of the healing treatment that they received. He was grateful for the blessing of Reiki and would also be grateful for their support. He would work with integrity each day. He would do his best. He would be compassionate and kind.

"The Reiki principles are not religious dogma or doctrine," practitioners are told. "These are not commandments." Instead, Reiki masters invite practitioners to reflect on Mrs. Takata's story of Dr. Usui and on the principles, and to remember them as aids to making healthy choices in their own lives: to choose to be calm instead of angry, relaxed rather than anxious, and always appreciative; to work with integrity for peace of mind and self-respect; and to be kind. Making these choices promotes mental, emotional, and spiritual health and well-being.

In Japan, where the Reiki principles have been well known in their more complete form to practitioners for generations, they're also deeply valued: practitioners recite the principles as a form of meditation, as Mikao Usui recommended. This means that twice daily, morning and night, with their hands joined in gassho, practitioners hear the double titles and register their promise of happiness and health; they repeat the five core statements and remind themselves that "just for today," they have the opportunity to choose peace, serenity, gratitude, integrity, and kindness. There's no sacred or healing value accorded to the words of the principles themselves, as practitioners of Indian yoga ascribe to such Sanskrit words as *"Om."* There's simply twice-daily recitation to reinforce the intentions the principles express.

Whether we casually reflect on the Reiki principles from time to time or make a ritual of reciting them morning and night, we eventually come to appreciate their practical value in facing the challenges of our own lives. We learn to apply them quickly, the same way that we apply our hands to an injury. Instead of reacting to difficult situations with aggressive anger or defensive blame, we make the choice to respond with calm. Rather than feeling overwhelmed by worry, we learn to catch ourselves before we get caught up in fear, to stop the stressful thoughts by reminding ourselves, "Just for today, do not worry." We breathe, relax, let go of the worry, and look for the good.

We become deliberately mindful of the blessings in life, reviewing them on waking, before sleep, and in between, whenever we want to claim gratitude's power to shift our moods from downcast to upbeat. Feeling empowered, caring, and cared for, we commit day by day, sometimes hour by hour, to do our best, and discover that we enjoy feeling good about our efforts. At peace with ourselves, we find that it's easy to be kind to others—and to ourselves. These many small changes in our way of thinking and behaving help us to feel harmony in mind and body, creating health and inviting happiness into our lives.

In Japan, there's one more way that the value of the Reiki principles is reinforced: before a *rei-ju,* or empowerment with the Reiki energy, the *shihan,* or Reiki master, invites the students who are to be attuned to join in a meditation on the Reiki principles. First, the Reiki master alone recites the principles aloud, and then the Reiki master and students recite the principles aloud together. Finally, everyone recalls the principles in silence. This suggests the power of the principles to transform our lives, even as the experience of the energy during an attunement transforms our hands.

SUMMARY

In the West and throughout much of the world, the Reiki principles have not been given as much attention as they deserve. Hawayo Takata, the twenty-two

Reiki masters she initiated, and later generations of Reiki masters teaching in the same tradition have presented the Reiki principles as spiritual precepts that Mikao Usui adopted for meditation as a consequence of his encounter with an ungrateful beggar. Even today, students who learn Usui Shiki Ryoho Reiki and hear about the Reiki principles for the first time are encouraged to simply reflect on them and remember them as they go about their daily lives. They're discouraged from thinking of them as doctrine or dogma.

Whether because Takata's telling of the story of Mikao Usui's life was informal or because her presentation of the Reiki principles included commentary, her students didn't always record them with the same wording or in the same sequence. The Reiki masters she initiated taught—and some continue to teach—their students in the same way as they learned from Takata. For this reason, there are still sometimes differences in the way traditional Reiki masters present the Reiki principles to their students.

In the 1990s, many people became more interested in making more accurate information about the early history of Reiki in Japan available worldwide. In Japan, German Reiki Master Frank Arjava Petter and his then wife, Chetna M. Kobayashi, attempted to learn more about the origins of Reiki. Japanese Reiki Master Hiroshi Doi came to the West to share information about how Reiki had been practiced and taught in Japan, with the approval of the Gakkai, the Reiki learning society founded during the time of Mikao Usui. In books and manuals, they published new and more complete translations of the Reiki principles, with the intriguing double title "The Secret Method of Inviting Happiness/The Miracle Medicine for All Diseases" given to them by "the Founder, Mikao Usui." Above his signature is the recommendation to recite the principles twice daily, morning and night, as a form of meditation.

Surely, the Reiki principles deserve to receive greater attention. Mikao Usui meditated upon them each day and regarded them as important tenets of his own spiritual practice. Whether we simply reflect upon them more often or adopt the practice of twice-daily recitation, we'll likely come to a deeper understanding of their place in Reiki practice. We may also discover that practice of the principles unleashes Reiki's power to bring healing into our lives in new and wonderful ways.

MORE SUGGESTIONS FOR PRACTICE

✤ Look over the various translations of the Reiki principles within this chapter. Which one do you prefer? Is it the one that's most familiar? Or is it one that is new to you but that makes emotional or spiritual sense? Consider experimenting with reciting a familiar version of the Reiki principles before you begin doing self-treatment or distant healing each day. Do you notice the energy coming into your hands as you say the principles? Let your experiment continue for several days. Do you have an easier time remembering the principles during the day?

✤ Sit or stand in a comfortable posture, with your hands in gassho: joined together, palm to palm, at the level of your heart. Read one of the more recent and complete translations of the Reiki principles, from the double title to the signature. Does this feel comfortable to you or unnatural and foreign? Do you notice the Reiki energy in your hands as you recite the principles? After briefly reciting the Reiki principles, practice hands-on or distant healing. At the end of the day, with your hands in gassho, repeat the recitation of the Reiki principles. Does this reminder of spiritual values seem a good way to

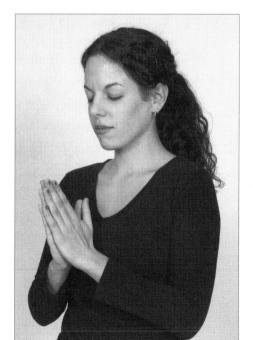

Gassho posture

bring closure to the day? Or does it seem too ritualized for your taste? Does it seem to quicken the flow of energy in your hands? Again, experiment with this practice for several days to get a sense of its power to affect your Reiki practice and the quality of your daily life.

✤ The principles are written in second-person viewpoint, as instructions or directions to "you," the student. When we recite them, we sound as if we're talking to ourselves. Yet Mikao Usui's signature, in the most complete translations, reminds us that these are instructions from the very first Reiki master, the founder. Does reciting the complete translation make Mikao Usui become more real and familiar to you? Do you feel encouraged to call upon him as a spiritual guide?

✤ In our culture, the use of affirmations has become popular as a way to bring about changes for the better in our lives. One of the keys to creating effective affirmations is to use the present tense and to frame each statement as a positive assertion, because the subconscious mind (we are told) doesn't understand the word *no*. Think about the first two Reiki principles, which are framed in the negative. Would you prefer "just for today, be at peace; just for today, be relaxed and calm . . ."? Or would you feel more comfortable with wording more typical of affirmations: "Just for today, I am peaceful, I am calm," and so on? The use of the present tense asserts that your positive intention is already reality—one of the reasons affirmations are considered so effective. Yet there is one more way you can reinforce your intention. Use the future tense: "Just for today, I will be peaceful, I will be calm, I will be grateful, I will do an honest day's work, I will be kind." Try out your own wording, affirming your intention to act according to the spiritual values that the principles recommend. See if you can discover a wording that resonates as true and meaningful for you and brings the energy strongly into your hands.

✤ The principles are conceptual tools for changing consciousness that have a very interesting relationship to the Reiki energy. Consider what else you might do on a daily or regular basis to become more mindful of the values they express: peace, serenity, gratitude, integrity, and kindness. As you involve yourself more actively with bringing these values into your life, do you sense the energy more? Do you feel healthier and happier? Record your impressions in a journal—and be honest. If you're disappointed that your life has changed less than you had hoped, there may be a reason for your resistance that you need to identify, some memory that needs to be recalled, released, and forgiven.

❧ In attempting to practice the Reiki principles and bring the values they express more fully into your life, you may, at times, feel acutely aware of your own need for mental, emotional, and spiritual healing. Remember that you can use Reiki hands-on and distant healing methods to address this need. For example, you can call in yourself as a client and offer Reiki to heal your quick temper, your habit of worrying, or your inability to forgive someone.

❧ If you're a teaching Reiki master, consider your own beliefs regarding the history of Reiki. Most of us are reluctant to abandon any way of thought that we've embraced as truth, even when researchers "enlighten" us by presenting us with the notes and journals of historical personages, legal documents, or period artifacts. Change is a constant, and adapting to change can be hard. Perhaps for that very reason, some Reiki masters in the Western (Usui Shiki Ryoho) tradition continue to teach the history of Reiki just as Takata told it, preserving it, despite some inaccuracies. Takata's account has historical value, and her story of the life of Mikao Usui can be appreciated for the many parable-like incidents that invite contemplation and offer both comfort and inspiration. Other Reiki masters in the Usui Shiki Ryoho tradition recount Takata's story of Mikao Usui's life and then describe the significant events in his life that are recorded on the Usui Memorial. Some have given up Takata's story altogether and provide only the more accurate historical account of Usui's life, while continuing to teach hand positions and to do attunements as their Takata-trained teachers taught them.

As a Reiki master, how will you now teach the history of Reiki? How will you present the Reiki principles? Will you invite your students to meditate on the principles before you attune them? Do you think you might place a greater emphasis on the Reiki principles than your own teacher did before you? Would you be comfortable encouraging your students to look at different translations of the principles to get a richer sense of their meaning and value in practice? Will you suggest that your students try reciting the principles daily? However you answer these questions, remember that the energy is the true teacher as well as the true healer. It does not judge us but flows through our hands for the purpose of healing, no matter which version of history we relate, no matter which translation of the principles we present.

PEACE

"Just for Today, Do Not Anger"

The Reiki principles begin with this simple recommendation: "Just for today, do not anger." Across the translations, the wording doesn't vary, making the interpretation straightforward. Today, moment by moment, don't react to violence with violence; don't respond to insults or barbs with cutting words; no matter how you're provoked, don't allow dark thoughts to arise and gather in your mind, like the threatening clouds that precede a storm. Do not anger. Of course, following this guidance is often easier said than done.

Beth Gray, my teacher for Reiki I and II, presented this principle with an added instruction: "Accept." This implies a possible next step: let go of any desire or attachment to a particular outcome or result; accept what is. This practice is in keeping with Buddhist philosophy now and in Japan when Reiki originated. Some practitioners can learn to retreat from anger into nonattachment and acceptance quickly and effectively, but those who were taught the Western values of creative problem solving and constructive action sometimes have problems with the passivity of this practice.

The original principle, however, does not advise acceptance or nonattachment. It stops short of telling us how to respond to anger-provoking situations and people. This leaves some of us wondering what behavior to choose. Are we being asked to be gentle in manner, to maintain peace of mind, and to remain calm, whatever challenges face us? I think so. I believe that, as channels of Reiki energy, as practitioners of the Reiki principles, we're being invited to choose peace: to become at peace with our lives and with our world, and to radiate peace wherever we go.

REIKI TEACHES PEACE

Reiki teaches us about peace, for as we "listen" to our hands, focusing our attention on the flow of energy, our thoughts slow and our minds become quiet. We have the opportunity to experience this peace whenever we take the time to do a complete treatment on ourselves or on a client: to be fully present to the energy, wholly aware of its gentleness, mindful of its healing power. Centered in the energy, surrendered to its flow, we become channels for peace. As we relax in response to the energy, we feel our own inner conflicts dissolve, and we observe our clients responding to Reiki in the same way: as they release physical tension, they let go of mental confusion and emotional turmoil. We become observers of the peace process on a very personal level, and as we learn to recognize the value of this evolution in ourselves and our clients, we become peacekeepers as well.

Simply by doing daily self-treatment, we promote our own inner peace, and by encouraging our clients to receive regular treatments and, in time, to learn Reiki, we promote peace in our world. How much further toward the goal of peace can the practice of the Reiki principles take us? Perhaps any conflict avoided or peacefully resolved is a battle won. If so, then the intention to refuse to anger "just for today" may take us far down the path toward inner peace and peace on earth.

Will we always be able to practice Reiki with this conscious awareness of its peaceful nature? No. If we treat our own or someone else's upset stomach, headache, sprain, or the like as we listen to the news on the radio, watch a colleague's presentation at work, or chauffeur the family to a baseball game, we aren't giving our complete attention to the flow of energy. Nor should we! We must claim a few minutes of quiet time in solitude to treat ourselves each day or devote an hour or two to treatment of a client to experience the Reiki energy's ability to bring us into our own peaceful center. Then, with an awareness of our own inner peace, we'll be better able to live our lives and to live *better* lives.

Committing to practice the Reiki principles each day quickens our healing and the evolution of our spiritual understanding and enlightenment. Soon, we feel determined to choose peace as a way of being. Instead of getting caught up in the rush of life as we sit down to work in a busy office or join the crowds at a shopping mall, we radiate a sense of well-being and harmony that touches those around us, quietly uplifting and inspiring them. Instead of feeling provoked by deliberate antagonism, frustrated by injustice, or infuriated by neglect, we remain calm and capable of constructive action. We embody peace, and on a soul level, because we are at peace, others know that peace is possible as well.

How does Reiki heal anger? Hands-on and distant healing can heal old anger that we've carried forward from the past, and it can diffuse anger in the present. Does remembering the Reiki principle "just for today, do not anger" work in the same way, dissolving long-standing enmity and calming us through today's moments of crisis? Is remembrance enough to help us let go of anger?

One day last fall, as I did distant healing, I connected to Dr. Usui and asked him to show me how to overcome the resistance and resentment—both of which are forms of anger—that I felt at the time. He showed me a small boulder placed squarely in the middle of my path. Then he waited for me to realize that I had three choices: I could beam Reiki energy at the boulder, which represented my negativity, and the energy would gradually dissolve it. I could avoid the boulder by choosing to walk around it and continuing on my way. Or I could reach down, lift up the boulder, and throw it out of my way.

I was fascinated by this guidance: I could use Reiki energy to dissolve the problem; I could choose not to focus on the problem at all, sidestep it, and continue forward; or I could face it and use whatever emotional management skills and wisdom I've gained as leverage to remove it from my path. The first method was familiar to me in the form of distant healing, and I knew it to be an excellent way to permanently resolve the problem.

Did the second method, deliberate avoidance, also offer an effective way of practicing Reiki, this time by following the recommendation of the first Reiki principle, "Just for today, do not anger"? This seemed a good possibility: I could look away from my negative feelings, just as if I were glancing away from a boulder in my path. I could focus instead on seeing where I could move forward. Then I could take the next obvious step, and then the next, and keep going until I was past this obstacle. This meant that I had to detach myself enough from those negative feelings that blocked my way that I would be able to see them as separate from me and not essential to my nature. This was appealing. I knew that as soon as I stopped fueling my own resistance and resentment with my attention, these negative feelings would start to lose their hold over me. I could retreat from my anger into acceptance and nonattachment. I would be in a better mood, in lighter spirits, energized, and free to go forward. And if for some reason I slipped again into a mindset of resistance and anger, I could go through the same process and make the same choice, repeating it as often as necessary to get past a particular emotional and mental obstacle to my progress.

The final image I was shown, that of lifting up the boulder and tossing it out of my way, was also intriguing. Did confronting and understanding the problem reduce its mass and weight enough that I could raise it up in my awareness and then set it aside? Did this represent another way to apply the first principle? Perhaps it did. I recalled Reiki Master Beth Gray, in class after class, emphasizing the importance of being willing to do the work of healing old, unresolved emotional problems, lest they become "stuck issues in the tissues." Was I being invited to reflect on these familiar negative feelings so that I could apply the light of my now more evolved consciousness, understand, and then forgive whatever circumstances and people in my past had fostered them? With this done, could I set aside any remaining negativity and go forward? This, too, seemed a valid way.

When I asked for and received this guidance about how to heal my feelings of anger, I didn't completely understand it, but I did feel compelled to continue to think about it. I recognized that, although I might not have a straightforward answer to my question, I did have Reiki-charged hands, the ability to recite and remember the Reiki principles, and a willingness to reflect on my life in order to identify the original source of my anger and then understand, forgive, and let go. Over the next few months, as I continued to direct Reiki toward this problem, practiced the Reiki principles each day, and consciously processed my feelings, I found that the resistance and resentment I had felt melted away. I feel grateful for the guidance, the healing, the lesson, and, more than ever before, committed to Reiki as pathwork.

REIKI:
THE MIRACLE MEDICINE FOR ANGER

Sometime in the late 1980s, as I assisted Reiki Master Beth Gray at a Reiki I class, I listened in astonishment as a student raged on about the prognosis her doctors had given her. This woman sat at the front of the class. She was beautiful, with long, blond waves of hair framing a delicate face and a slender figure. She wore an elegant business suit that did nothing to hide her paralyzed legs, supported by the sturdy brackets of a wheelchair.

"I was in a car accident earlier this year," she said. "The doctors told me I will never walk again." Then her voice became loud and brittle with bitterness: "They say I will *never* walk again! Are you telling me that Reiki will make some kind of difference? How could it?"

Beth said quietly, "Just give Reiki a chance. Just try it."

The woman seemed outraged by these simple words, but Beth remained calm, and eventually the woman responded by becoming calm herself.

Although I didn't have the chance to meet this woman during her level I class, about ten years later, I saw her again, at a gathering of some of Beth Gray's students in 1998. She was still as beautiful as ever. She stood tall and walked gracefully, without even the use of a cane. She had continued to use Reiki during all the intervening years, and she had become a Reiki master.

When Melissa Flowers first contacted me, she told me that she was interested in receiving Reiki treatments and perhaps in learning Reiki to help her to cope with on-the-job stress and tension. At her first session, she explained that she worked in the bookkeeping department of a local manufacturing company, and she was tired of her gossipy, backbiting colleagues, especially their leader. Every workday, as Melissa sat at her desk in the cubicle she shared with them, she endured the hostile atmosphere in silence and refused to participate. This made her an occasional target of their snipes. As she received regular Reiki treatments over a period of a couple months, she realized that the gentle healing energy relaxed her very deeply. Her troubles seemed to fade away, and she remained unaffected by them until the next morning, when she returned to work and had to face her coworkers again.

After receiving a few Reiki treatments, Melissa decided to learn Reiki. Yet she continued to come for regular client treatments every few weeks, because she desired that very deep relaxation. One workday evening, after she greeted me and caught me up on how she was doing, she told me that she had made a decision: "Tomorrow morning, I'm going to say something to that woman to silence her once and for all. I've had enough of her and all of them. I don't want to spend eight hours every day in such a poisonous atmosphere. I can't take it anymore. I've figured out exactly what I'm going to tell her to put a stop to this."

I nodded, at a loss for a comment. I encouraged her to put down her purse on a chair and lie down on the bodywork table, which was prepared for her, covered with fresh linens and a pillow. I proceeded to do a complete hands-on Reiki treatment. I gave particular attention to her lower rib cage area on the front of her body, high above the adrenal glands, and to her midsection, where the solar plexus chakra is located. In both areas, the Reiki energy flow was very strong in response to her extreme level of stress. During the course of the treatment, she became visibly more relaxed. When I had completed all the standard positions, front, head, and back, I invited her to roll over in a face-up position again. Then I worked in her energy field, letting my hands follow the familiar pattern, listening to the energy to determine when to shift position. In her energy field, the flow of the Reiki energy seemed even more intense.

When I had treated her field thoroughly, I asked, "Melissa, how do you feel?"

She smiled slowly, "I feel wonderful." Then she paused, "But there's only one problem—"

I frowned at this unexpected response. "What's that?" I asked.

"I don't feel like saying anything to that woman at work anymore. It's as if all my determination to set things straight just dissolved." She sighed.

Again, I wasn't sure how to comment. "Well, that's interesting . . . ," I said, letting my voice drift off.

About a month later, when Melissa came for another treatment, she greeted me with a bright smile. "You'll never guess what's happened at work!" she said. "I've been transferred to another department, one where I really like my coworkers, and I like what I'm doing better than before. I can't believe it! And I never said a word to that woman—and I didn't put in a transfer request."

I thought about how this problem had led Melissa to seek me out for Reiki treatments and then motivated her to learn Reiki. I nodded. "I think that's the Reiki energy at work, shifting your situation a bit to enhance the quality of your life. I think perhaps you've just had your first Reiki miracle."

NOW YOU: USE REIKI IN THE ENERGY FIELD TO DISSOLVE ANGER

Using Reiki in the energy field is a powerful way to heal habitual negative thoughts and feelings. Reiki Master Beth Gray sometimes recommended this technique in her classes for dealing with chronic conditions accompanied by depression or other "stuck" emotions. She considered it particularly effective in healing negative thoughts and feelings that have been repeated so often that they reinforce tiredness, sickness, sadness—whatever the complaint. So the next time you feel frustrated, resentful, infuriated, or annoyed—whether the catalyst is the memory of a past event, a pattern of negative thinking first triggered by a past event, or some difficulty in the present, try using Reiki in your own energy field. Even sitting at a desk chair, you can float your hands in front of your heart to heal sadness and sorrow. Or you can float one hand in front of your heart and another in front of your navel, at the level of the solar plexus chakra, to calm emotions that have to do with the will and the sense of gaining or losing control, such as anger, shame, humiliation, hurt, and anxiety.

Don't wait until you're faced with a situation that arouses your fury or provokes a panic attack. Try this experiment when you feel mildly frustrated or annoyed, or when you realize that your thoughts hold whispers of worry. Find out now how effective this technique can be in restoring your tranquility, so that you'll immediately remember to use it in crisis.

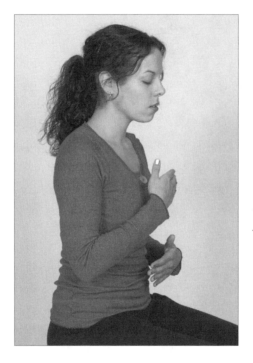

Work in your energy field over your heart and solar plexus to bring quick relief from anger and frustration.

Once you feel comfortable using this technique on yourself and confident of its effectiveness, consider offering it to clients who walk into the Reiki treatment session carrying the emotional baggage of old anger or worry. It's equally valuable for clients who have been fighting or arguing, and those who are anxious about some current concern. A good way to proceed is to do a complete hands-on Reiki treatment and then follow up with work in the energy field. You might focus on the client's heart and solar plexus chakras only; float your hands above the client's body in a pattern corresponding to your standard hand positions; or move slowly through the client's energy field, stopping wherever the sensations in your hands become more active and intense, and staying until they become quiet. All of these techniques will help your client to heal both old, smoldering angers, and irritation and annoyance at today's injustices. An interesting side effect of working in the client's energy field after a complete hands-on treatment is that all of the healing that occurs in the physical body seems to take a deeper hold and have even more lasting benefits.

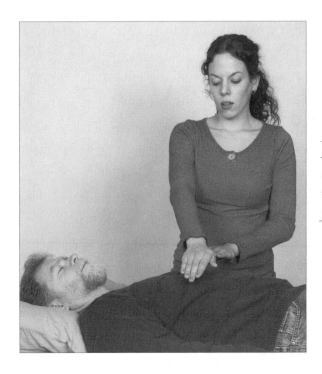

At the completion of a client treatment, do additional Reiki in the client's energy field to facilitate more lasting healing.

HAWAYO TAKATA'S REFUSAL TO ANGER

Hawayo Takata had a reputation for having a temper. Whether or not that reputation is deserved, she made every effort to live by the Reiki principles. In her book *Living Reiki: Takata's Teachings,* Takata-initiated Reiki Master Fran Brown tells of Takata's encounters with Sadie, a woman who took repeated advantage of her kindness, begging money from her again and again. Takata responded to the woman's distress and helped her by giving her money for the passage home from Japan to Hawaii, for business creditors so she could leave her affairs in good order, and even for weekly household expenses in Hawaii, when the woman reported that her husband refused to give her money even for necessities.

Finally, Sadie came to Takata to ask her for money for the fare back to

Japan. Takata gave it to her gladly, thinking it a worthwhile price to pay to end this relationship. A few hours later, however, Sadie returned to beg the cost of the fare again, saying that she had spent the earlier gift of money on clothes to refresh her wardrobe for the trip to Japan. The story continues:

> This was the last straw! Takata was furious!
>
> She returned to Dr. Hayashi and said, "This, this, this, this, this thing that is happening . . . can I get mad just this one time? . . . I just want to use my elbow grease and give her a punch in the eye and knock her down the stairs so she can't come back any more!"
>
> Hayashi said, "If you fly off the handle you will be hurting yourself. So do not anger." He smiled and turned the other way.
>
> Takata took a deep breath and told herself, "I will not anger today." Very gently, she said to Sadie, "Do you see that doorway, and the veranda beyond, and the six steps down to the walkway? Please go down there and out the gate, and never come back to me again. I have no ears to hear you."
>
> Takata was determined to live by the Reiki ideals.[1]

When Takata calmly told Sadie to leave and never to return, she established a firm, protective boundary around herself. When she told Sadie that her pleas would not be heard, Takata ended an abusive relationship. However, this was not the last of Sadie, who promised revenge as she walked away. Sadie made a false report to the U.S. Department of Immigration officials that Hayashi and Takata were in the United States illegally and that they were charging money for lectures and demonstrations advertised in newspapers as free to the public. Hayashi was interviewed by an immigration officer and had to show his passport, visa, and traveler's checks. When the official saw that Hayashi's documents were entirely in order and he carried ample cash with him for all his own and his family's needs, the official apologized for the misunderstanding. Yet the difficulties were not quite over: policemen were posted outside the lecture hall where Hayashi spoke about Reiki to stop those leaving and ask whether or not they had been charged money for the lecture or their "consultation." Of course, they had not.

When the story came out in the newspapers, it aroused a lot of sympathy for the Hayashi family and for Takata so that the lecture halls were filled up with even more people who were interested in learning about Reiki. Perhaps because of the power of Reiki to heal difficult situations or because of Takata's determined application of the Reiki principle, "Just for today, do not anger," Sadie's revenge backfired. Rather than damaging Hayashi's or Takata's reputation, Sadie gained them many supporters; and instead of forcing the Hayashis out of Hawaii, a congressional delegate assured Takata that they could ". . . stay through February, the limit of their visas."[2]

NOW YOU: REFUSE TO ANGER

Anger can build into an emotional firestorm, especially when fueled by two people who are willing to keep giving it their conscious attention. When one person stops attending to the fire, by ignoring it or deliberately walking away, the one remaining has to work much harder to keep the blaze going. With Hayashi's encouragement, Takata made the decision to live by the principle, "Just for today, do not anger." Deliberately, she cooled down her feelings in a difficult, frustrating situation and, instead, found a way to resolve and end it. Sadie's response of fury proved futile, and her retaliation failed. Why? It certainly seems as if Takata's remembrance of the Reiki principles invited Reiki energy to flow to the situation and bring about the healing that was for the highest good of all concerned.

If you are quick to anger, allow yourself to be inspired by Takata's courage and commitment to Reiki. Make the decision to recite the Reiki principles each day. Remind yourself not to anger but to choose peace. Throughout the day, refuse to anger. This may require that you walk away from situations that make you feel outraged or from individuals who bait you. This will take courage and may require inner strength since patience, determination, and real effort are often necessary to contain and reduce such intense emotions. Realize, too, that the first time you refuse to anger in such a situation, you may feel that instead of making a moral or wise choice, you're a coward running away from "a good fight." Don't be fooled by years of past cultural conditioning. There are always better ways to resolve problems than fighting or going to war. Look for constructive solutions, and until they appear, use Reiki distant healing to dissolve the obstacles.

What if you cannot walk away? What if you feel you *must* stay in the job long enough to collect your pension or in the relationship because of the children? If you're unwilling to walk away, then at least learn how to avoid adding fuel to the fire of anger. Learn to withdraw your emotional energy and refocus your attention on some healthier, happier aspect of your life. Find some way to go forward, even if it means avoiding the anger-provoking situation or person for now. This is not the same as denying that a problem exists. To withdraw your emotional energy and attention from a troubling situation, you have to acknowledge it and recognize how much it drains and depletes you. Then you can see it with more objectivity, detach from it, and consider how to move forward.

HEALING THE PAST TO MOVE FORWARD IN THE PRESENT

Sometimes difficult situations in the present seem echoes of the past. This can occur when the past situation has never been fully resolved, the emotional wounds never healed, and the individuals involved never forgiven. A single traumatic event, such as an assault or robbery or rape, can result in this kind of psychological and spiritual pain, but having to cope with ongoing difficulties, such as an alcoholic or verbally abusive parent or partner, can also create emotional wounds that are difficult to heal.

For this reason, when I teach Reiki II, besides inviting students to practice sending distant healing to an unknown client, to themselves, to the earth, and to one of the early Reiki teachers, I also ask if anyone would like the class as a group to send healing forward in time or back in time, to an event that was traumatic in some way. Often, a student will volunteer that he or she has suffered from abuse and would like help in healing old emotional wounds. This is a very positive step toward complete healing.

In order for us to become whole and enjoy health and happiness, we must be willing to heal the past and to find a way that brings us a sense of closure. Although we must accept that we cannot change the past, we can use Reiki to lessen its hold over us. Being freed of shame, guilt, anger, or depression that's

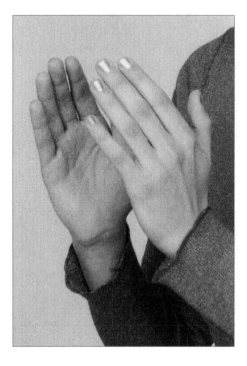

Practice Reiki distant healing to become familiar with the symbols and method so that you can apply it to bring healing in many ways, including sending it back in time.

rooted in decades-old trauma can make a dramatic difference in the quality of our lives, enabling us to be at peace with ourselves and to reclaim a strong sense of self-worth. While this healing is usually a gradual process, once it begins, we may find ourselves taking pleasure in the present moment more and more often. This, too, restores and refreshes us. Healed, at peace, and empowered, we discover that our positive attitude attracts even greater good.

Psychiatrists tell us that violent crimes are not about passion but about power. While it's completely appropriate to fight off perpetrators of such crimes, few victims are able to do so. They're left with not only a sense of violation and shame but also a guilty awareness of their own lack of strength. Since perpetrators are often familiar to the victims, guilt is compounded by confusion: what has happened to love or friendship, and affection? If this individual cannot be trusted to care, can anyone? If relatives are unwilling to listen to an account or to believe in the reality of the crime, shame and self-doubt intensify. Without proper counseling, serious depression often sets in, and the struggle to overcome it can go on for years, even for a lifetime.

Reiki can, indeed, heal depression over time, and it can also heal feelings of guilt, shame, self-doubt, and self-loathing. One of the most effective ways to bring about this healing is by a committed effort to send Reiki back in time. Whether we send it to ourselves or a client, Reiki can bring healing and release from the spiritual and emotional impact of traumatic events.* Reiki can also complement crisis counseling, psychotherapy, hypnosis, and the various forms of art therapy, which all help the individual to move forward into healthier relationships with others and a healthier sense of self.

Is such healing always necessary? It is certainly possible to live a good, moral life without reviewing the details of a painful past, but happiness and fulfillment are likely to remain elusive unless the need for healing on all levels is addressed in some way. As for attaining spiritual wisdom and peace of mind, is this possible for anyone who is at war with ghosts? We must learn to forgive the past, to forgive those who have injured us, and to forgive ourselves if we hope to move forward with our lives.

Addiction and addictive behavior patterns, which are usually rooted in the past, can also be treated successfully with Reiki, particularly when Reiki is used as complementary medicine. As much as society celebrates the ideal of a happy childhood, few of us manage to survive to adulthood without having to negotiate some fairly treacherous emotional waters along the way. Alcoholism, drug addiction, problems with debt or gambling, illness and unemployment, marital difficulties and divorce, can all cause the stable family, so important to the development of healthy children, to become unstable and dysfunctional. In order to "fix" the broken family, many children go through a process of recognizing that they can't change mom or dad, so they must change themselves to keep the family intact. They may accept various enabler or codependent roles, including those of caretaker or peacemaker. They may attempt to rebalance the family by becoming underachievers or overachievers, or struggling for

---

*Traditionally taught (Usui Shiki Ryoho) Reiki incorporates a permission step into the distant-healing method, rather than requiring the practitioner to seek the client's conscious permission, as some more modern forms of Reiki instruction do. The wording of the permission step might be as follows: "I offer you Reiki healing. You are free to accept or to reject it for your own highest good and the highest good of all concerned." This acknowledgment of the client's free will and release of the outcome are considered sufficient in terms of seeking client permission, and it is understood that healing will be accepted or rejected on a soul level. This allows the practitioner to offer Reiki distant healing more broadly than might otherwise be possible, including to people with whom the practitioner is no longer in contact, for example, the perpetrators of long-ago abuse or domestic violence, a drug-addicted parent, or an alcoholic ex-spouse.

mediocrity to escape all attention. At some point, they may blame themselves for the family's problems and become self-destructive but then later reverse this by casting blame on the parents and acting out in anger.

The problem with developing such unhealthy coping patterns in childhood is that they often endure into adulthood. If a behavior works once, it's repeated; if it works often, it becomes a habitual coping style. Children who develop such patterns to survive in dysfunctional family environments grow into adults who are prepared for more dysfunction, and they tend to have difficulty forming long-lasting, loving relationships with healthy partners.

Reiki can help to heal these old emotional wounds as well. Distant healing, directed back in time can help to heal the hurt, angry inner child who still exists in repressed memories and who often hides within the heart and mind of the mature adult. Practicing the Reiki principles can also offer a way to form new, healthy patterns of behavior. Remembering the first principle, "Just for today, do not anger," can be as helpful as finding the oars in a boat that's out of control, floating downstream in a fast current toward the rapids.

If you or someone you know is interested in healing old, unhealthy patterns of behavior, rather than using Reiki alone, consider it complementary medicine to counseling and mental health support groups, such as Alcoholics Anonymous, Adult Children of Alcoholics, Narcotics Anonymous, and the like. Making an effort to learn more about child development in dysfunctional families, anger management, and healthy communication skills may also be of benefit. Increased knowledge and understanding can offer a foundation for positive change. Renowned authors John Bradshaw, Melody Beattie, and Harriet Lerner have written books on healing the inner child, codependency, and anger, respectively, which are clear and accessible to lay readers. In particular, Harriet Lerner's groundbreaking book, *The Dance of Anger: A Woman's Guide to Changing the Patterns of Intimate Relationships,* teaches readers to acknowledge responsibility for feelings rather than to cast or take blame. The examples she presents demonstrate how setting clear boundaries and learning improved communication skills can help people who grew up in dysfunctional families to become healthy adults, freed from anger and capable of leading fulfilling lives.

REPEAT "JUST FOR TODAY, I WILL NOT ANGER"

Since 1998, John Connors has worked as a warehouse manager, receiving shipments from vendors and scanning them into inventory, in grocery stores owned by three separate chains. Although he prefers to stay at one location, he has been transferred five times. When he works in a newly opened store, it's well staffed for about the first six months to build up customer loyalty, and then the workforce is cut to economize. John's role is essential, however, and he knows how to perform his responsibilities well, so he has never been laid off. His underpaid coworkers are often asked to work extended hours without overtime, so there's a lot of turnover—and a lot of dissatisfaction.

John has a strong sense of integrity, and for many years, has tried to do his best to keep the warehouse he runs in good order and always inspection ready. More and more often, though, when he clocks in at 6:30 a.m., he has to pick up after the night crew, who leave crushed cardboard boxes and discarded pallets strewn around the warehouse floor. He doesn't like this job, because it *isn't* his job. It's the night crew's responsibility to clean up after themselves. Sometimes, depending on how he finds the condition of the warehouse, he feels himself becoming angry.

To avoid becoming angry, he has learned to prepare for the day by getting up at 4:30 a.m., and taking time to meditate and pray. He thinks about what he will probably face on the job and reminds himself that he's not responsible for the working conditions that have created an indifferent workforce. He tells himself that he is responsible for the warehouse but only on his watch. He reminds himself not to get angry, to count to ten, to breathe, to use the Reiki symbols, and to practice the Reiki principles—and then he goes in to work.

Every day, something comes up to try his patience. "I figure I'm here to learn how to do the best I can in a difficult situation and be okay with it," he says. "Each day, I start out with the intention that I'm not going to anger. I'm going to stay calm. I'm going to choose peace. I figure that I must still be learning that lesson or I would be working at a different job, in a different place." Besides focusing on remembering the Reiki principles, John has made the choice to see his place of employment as a kind of spiritual testing ground.

Because he's aware that he'll be challenged throughout the day to remain faithful to his values, he reflects on his responses afterward, understands the lessons, and claims his own spiritual growth.

NOW YOU: SEE YOUR SITUATION IN A SPIRITUAL CONTEXT

One way to avoid feeling caught up in anger or overwhelmed by worry is to understand your problems in a spiritual context. Although a challenge you face today may evoke aggression or defensiveness in you, if you can see it as one brief episode in your life's journey, you may feel less tempted to lash out in rage or recoil in pain. It is but a moment, an hour, a day—a short span of time—that you will feel so preoccupied. Can you step back, take a breath, calm down, and see this event with a longer range perspective? Can you make a conscious decision to withdraw your attention and energy from the emotional drama and see yourself as separate from your feelings of anger and negativity? Perhaps you can—and as soon as you do, you'll be able to find a way to move on.

Here's a way to reenvision a situation that lessens its power to evoke anger or worry: reflect on it with the determination to see everything in it that is positive and good. Practice gratitude. Look for every blessing. Appreciate the smallest opportunity for constructive action. Praise the possibility of hope. Anticipate the spiritual lessons you'll learn. Be glad for the chance to be compassionate, kind, and understanding. And what if this feels difficult? Keep going. Gratitude is a different energetic state than anger—higher, finer, and lighter. You can move into that energetic state by choice and by doing the work, making the effort to withdraw your attention from whatever makes you angry and give your attention to whatever seems good. This is spiritual pathwork. When you find yourself smiling more often and enjoying moments of peace, you'll know that you've moved past the anger. Keep going. Keep practicing gratitude for your life's blessings. You're on your way.

LIFE LESSONS ON PLANET EARTH

Life experience can teach us a great deal about anger and its management: On my first job out of college, I worked as a secretary in the rental office of a suburban high-rise building. My boss, a lawyer, was a perfectionist. One afternoon, I typed some letters for his signature and deposited them in his in-box. A few minutes later, he called me into his office. With one hand, he thrust a letter toward me and, with the other, pointed at a typographical error with his index finger. With cold fury, he said, "When I saw that typo, I was so angry, I wanted to strangle you." Since his anger seemed way out of proportion to my mistake, I remained calm and said, "I'm sorry. It won't happen again." His scowl deepened. His voice rose a few decibel levels. He shouted, "When I saw that, I was so angry, I wanted to strangle you!" Now I realized that there must have been something more than the transposition of two letters on a typed page that made him angry. I had been elected scapegoat. I stayed calm, and I repeated my apology, "I'm sorry. It won't happen again." His face reddened with fury. He repeated his threat one more time, even more loudly—and I kept my voice level and apologized once more. Then he sighed, like a balloon deflating. I knew his anger had dissipated. "All right," he said. "Get back to work."

This experience helped me realize that there are some situations in which anger can be diffused. When anger directed at you seems inappropriate or excessive, don't take it personally. Listen and hear what's being said, but remain calm. Keep your own tone of voice at a normal level. Accept responsibility for your mistakes, but don't allow yourself to be antagonized or intimidated. If you resist being caught up in an escalating cycle of anger, if you're willing to claim neutral ground, you can diffuse your attacker's anger altogether. This is one of the potential benefits of practicing the first principle: by refusing to anger, you may dissipate the anger of those around you. By your calm acceptance, you invite others to find inner calm.

Years later, a similar on-the-job experience reinforced this lesson. One summer, I worked as a temporary secretary in the office of the president of a manufacturing company. My boss was Italian, and his looks reminded me of my grandfather, a man with a volatile temper. When my boss raised his voice to me for the first time (when I lost a transatlantic phone call), I physically stepped back out of his reach. Seeing this, he found other reasons to raise his voice to me. He was entertained by my reaction to his bullying, but I caught on quickly. From then on, I remained calm and stood my ground. Our relationship became calm and productive as well. When I completed the three-week assignment, I was told that I would be welcomed back whenever a need arose.

Both of these experiences—one before and one after I learned Reiki—helped me understand the value of remaining calm in the face of another's anger, but I was by no means done with "life lessons" on anger management. For about ten years I lived in Philadelphia, where I received one parking ticket after another. Each time I received one I would rage inwardly at the unfairness of the ticket or the size of the fine or my own foolishness in letting the meter expire. I waited to pay the ticket until the last possible day, unwilling to give the city's parking authority my money a moment too soon. Sometimes, I even ended up paying an additional fine because I had waited too long to pay the ticket. Often, on the same day that I paid the parking ticket, I would discover that I had received another.

Eventually, tired of prolonged drain on my finances and the nearly constant undercurrent of anger that coursed through me, I thought about my problem in metaphysical terms. What had I ever done to attract so many parking tickets into my life? I soon realized that my hours and days of indulgence in anger on receipt of each parking ticket were as good as a written invitation to the universe to send me more. I resolved to change my ways: to say "thank you" for the lesson I was learning the next time I glimpsed a parking ticket under my windshield wiper; to stay calm and composed as I removed it and read the citation; to pay the ticket, if possible, within the hour; and then to forgive myself, the meter maid, and the situation—and let it all go. I promised myself to repeat this behavior for as long as necessary to change my negative thoughts and feelings into positive ones. Within a short time, there was a radical decline in the number of parking tickets I received.

This was a very practical lesson in the metaphysics of attraction. When we give the energy of our attention to something, it increases its importance in our lives. When we allow ourselves to become angry about a situation or event, we make it more important, and we tend to attract more situations or events like it into our lives. Sometimes we can find no single cause for our anger. Instead, we experience one minor annoyance after another until anger builds within us to dangerous, stressful levels. How can we resist lashing out in fury when we feel so continually confronted by the world? The trick is not to give undue attention to what annoys or irritates us. If we dwell on what frustrates or infuriates us, we fuel the fire of our own anger and, in consequence, we attract more that angers us into our lives.

NOW YOU:
APPLY THE LAW OF ATTRACTION

Reflect on the lessons you have learned about anger management in your own life. Can you recall an encounter where your choice to remain calm diffused another's anger? Can you remember an experience in which your refusal to be continually intimidated or bullied enabled you to stand your ground, maintain your self-respect, and say what needed to be said? Perhaps an experience with something breaking or being interrupted or delayed taught you to remain calm and patient and to persevere without complaint. Every lesson you have understood in the school of life is hard-earned knowledge. Remember what you have learned when anger tests you.

Remember, too, that you can apply the law of attraction to attract greater good. If you want to attract greater calm, peace, and harmony into your life, choose to remain calm and at peace even when confronted or challenged. Make this choice again and again: "Just for today, do not anger." Your focused attention on the principles and your dedication to Reiki healing practice will draw more positive-thinking, peaceful people into your life. You will see changes for the better in your world.

HEALING A COMMUNITY AFTER
A CRIME SPREE

Reiki Master Anna Desco is someone who believes that Reiki can bring peace and world healing. She cares passionately about the environment and has spent much of her life working for wildlife conservation organizations. She sends Reiki to the earth every day, including to the small Southern town in which she lives, where there is still some racial tension and distinct socioeconomic divisions.

Last summer, a string of robberies occurred in the town over a few weeks' time, bringing into sharp focus the need for healing within the community. As more and more homes were burglarized, many of the townspeople began living in fear and hiding behind their own closed doors. As the fifth, sixth, and seventh homes were burglarized, the news made the front page of the local paper—and Anna began sending Reiki distant healing to the situation in earnest. She also began asking Reiki friends to join her in sending healing to the situation.

Then, when she and her family went on a vacation, the burglar struck one more time. Anna and her husband and children came home to a picked lock, broken glass, and tossed drawers. The strange thing was that the only items stolen were of little value—loose change and her husband's childhood coin collection, which had personal and sentimental value to him rather than any monetary worth.

Anna and her husband were able to talk to each other and to their children about the sense of violation and loss they all felt. However, they also realized that the burglary wasn't personally directed at them but was indicative of a divided community's deep need for healing. Anna decided to do some meditation and ask for guidance about the situation. She contacted me to ask that the town be placed on a distant-healing list so that even more Reiki would be sent to the situation. Within a couple of days the burglar was caught, and Anna learned that he had mental health problems. She began to send distant healing to him regularly, which helped her begin the process of forgiveness, fueled by compassion.

This event, like most challenges, posed an opportunity for growth, and Anna decided she could no longer ignore what was happening in her community. She would become more involved. She formed a group of concerned citizens dedicated to providing a meeting place where parents and children from all the neighborhoods in the town can come together and experience their connection to each other, to their community, and to the earth in fun and innovative ways. She also plans to offer Reiki at this location.

She believes that resolving this crisis has forced the townspeople to reach out to one another in a way that they could not have before. While she knows that there is still an ongoing need for healing support, tensions have diminished, and she feels safer and more secure walking down her street as her neighbors call "hello" and stop to chat with her. She has great hope now that her town is on its way to becoming a strong, healthy community.

NOW YOU: HONOR DIVERSITY

Prejudice is one of the most painful wounds that one human being can inflict upon another. It falls as heavy as a club on the back of the head, and it slowly forces down those who do not stumble or fall immediately under its weight. While most Reiki practitioners and teachers feel a natural abhorrence to racism and other forms of social intolerance, there is one form we must carefully guard against in ourselves.

In the last two decades—which have seen the arrival on Western shores of Japanese Reiki masters with different techniques and a different history of Reiki—the global Reiki community has become more tolerant, open-minded, and appreciative of other traditions and cultures. Yet many Reiki practitioners and masters still judge and condemn their colleagues who have been taught or who teach in a different way, if not with outright statements then by silent criticism and censure. They use pride in their own way of doing Reiki as an excuse to set themselves above or apart from others on this path—an expression of intolerance that is divisive and damaging to global consciousness. This slows world healing.

While it is wise to use the highest possible spiritual discrimination when deciding where and when and how to learn Reiki and to ask for guidance in choosing a teacher, it is unwise to walk the path of Reiki forever guarding and defending the particular form of Reiki you have learned. It is also unwise to use the particular form in which you have received this spiritual gift to humanity to set yourself apart from or above others who walk the same path.

One of Reiki's most profound and humbling lessons is that the energy is the healer; another is that the energy is the teacher. When we recognize and reflect on the truth that Reiki is Spirit-guided life-force energy, we eventually come to realize that it is without limits or boundaries. It is everywhere we go and in everyone we meet. This realization can help us set aside preconceived judgments so that we may listen to others in the Reiki community in an open-minded, appreciative way that honors the energy in them. When we apply this lesson in our relationships with other Reiki practitioners and teachers we heal the Reiki community worldwide and help to accelerate world healing.

Reflect on your past and present relationships with fellow Reiki practitioners and teachers. Have you felt the weight of prejudice fall on your shoulders? Be kind. Forgive. Mentally, thank the individuals involved for the lessons and reclaim your sense of integrity and wholeness by doing Reiki; if you are an advanced practitioner, send Reiki back in time to the incidents to release yourself from their hold over you.

Consider also your own behavior. Has selfishness or arrogance predisposed you to judge or prevented you from listening with an open mind to another practitioner taught in a different way? Cast out false pride. Release the ego's attachment to the form of instruction with which you identify. Forgive yourself. Use Reiki to heal yourself. Go deeper into the energy that is unconditional love.

THE PLACE OF FORGIVENESS

While the first Reiki principle advises us not to anger, it doesn't offer any single solution to the problem of anger. We may refuse to become angry in a single, decisive moment, as Takata did when badly treated; we may contemplate the same decision over time, meditating on the principles and being mindful of them each day; or we may send Reiki healing into the past to heal old hurts, into the present to resolve problematic situations without antagonism, and into the future to invite peace.

In our practice of Reiki, where is the place of forgiveness? Sometimes in Reiki II classes, students asked Reiki Master Beth Gray if it was necessary to send Reiki to people they disliked or resented. Her answer, delivered with a warm smile and an approving nod of her head, was always the same: "Send Reiki to your enemies." Forgiveness, she told us, would help us to heal ourselves and all our relationships. It would free us from the bondage of the past so that we could move forward.

Forgiveness goes beyond mere avoidance of anger, or quiet acceptance of difficult circumstances or trying people. It allows for the possibility of conflict resolution through problem solving and constructive action to end aggression, but it doesn't stop there. Forgiveness takes the next step. Forgiveness enables us to let go of painful memories and set aside present fears without knowing the result of surrender. Forgiveness exhibits a generosity of spirit, a willingness to end the fighting for no other reason than a desire for peace. Forgiveness offers kindness to the person who was an enemy yesterday in order to bring closure and healing in the present and to claim the possibility of peace.

"I HAVE A WEAPON IN MY HANDS, AND THAT IS REIKI"

Ikechukwu Omenka was a schoolboy during the Biafran War (1967–70), which devastated Nigeria, taking the lives of a hundred thousand soldiers and causing the starvation of over two million civilians. His memories of this time in his life are so painful that he's reluctant to speak about it. Perhaps he remembers waking in the night to the sounds of shouting and machine gunfire or the thunder of bombs exploding nearby. Maybe he recalls seeing the slain bodies of "soldiers," who were children no older than he. These were common events.

Whatever he heard and saw was so traumatic to him that he ceased to be able to learn. He could no longer read the words on a printed page and comprehend them. He couldn't think clearly or write. For a time, he tried to overcome his fears by "crossing over to the enemy": he deliberately visited schoolmates whose families were from another tribe or religion. However, this wasn't enough to heal the cultural rifts that existed in the town where he lived, and it wasn't enough to heal his own grief and anguish at the war zone his country had become. Finally, his family sent him to Europe so that he could recover and continue his education.

Decades passed, and Ikechukwu eventually became an engineer. He stayed away from Nigeria, which, despite some political and economic recovery, was still plagued by tribal disputes, religious riots, and government appropriation of native lands. He didn't want to go back to his homeland, where so many families still lived in poverty and grieved the loss of parents, uncles, and sons.

Then, in 1991 he heard about the Reiki natural method of healing and decided that he was interested in it enough to travel from Austria, where he now lived and worked, to Germany to take a class. His teacher, Ursula Klinger-Raatz, had been trained as a Reiki master by Phyllis Furumoto, granddaughter of Hawayo Takata. Ikechukwu was grateful to learn Reiki, and remained in touch with his teacher, keeping her apprised of the healing that he experienced. So it wasn't a great surprise to her when he told her that he had decided to return to Nigeria with some of his fellow Reiki practitioners.

She asked if she might travel with the group, knowing that they were on a mission to observe conditions in the country and consider ways that they could bring about peace. He welcomed her to the group. So it was that they traveled together through Nigeria, visiting villages from north to south, meditating with others in the group to ask for guidance on how to help the people. In this way, the idea of a Reiki clinic in Nigeria was born. Near Ikechukwu's village, Ursula initiated everyone to Reiki II. Here, too, Ikechukwu and Ursula realized that they had fallen in love.

All too soon, the group flew home to Europe and to the routine of their daily lives, but Ikechukwu and Ursula made plans to return to Nigeria in 1992 to be married in a traditional ceremony and to break ground for the clinic to be built. Using their own funds, they purchased a sizeable plot of land out-side Avu, a village near Owerri in southwestern Nigeria. Hiring local workers and pitching in themselves, they began building a two-story, twenty-four-room building.

A year later, on their return to Überlingen, Germany, Ursula Klinger-Omenka initiated Ikechukwu as a Reiki master. Together, they worked at a holistic center they had established in Nonnenhorn, Germany, offering Reiki treatments and classes. In addition, Ikechukwu taught drumming, and Ursula taught workshops on the use of Reiki with crystals and semiprecious stones, the subject of one of her books, *Reiki with Gemstones*. Ikechukwu remembers this as "one of the happiest times" in his life.

Yet neither forgot their commitment to build a Reiki clinic in Nigeria. Year after year, they returned to supervise construction, to plant gardens and landscape, and to hire a permanent staff. On each visit, they taught Reiki and offered Reiki treatments to bring healing. However, before the clinic could open its doors, they found that they had run out of personal funds. They asked for support from European friends and found that this eliminated the shortfall.

In July 1999, the Reiki Clinic admitted its first clients on a token-fee or barter basis. Unfortunately, their Nigerian clients were poor and unable to pay even the small amount asked, and the idea of barter was unfamiliar to them. In addition, many of the clients needed allopathic care, which was provided by a doctor who stopped by the clinic once a week. The Omenkas found themselves paying for this service out of their own funds, so from the first, the clinic was not a moneymaking proposition. Then a preacher in a nearby Christian church started speaking out against the clinic and urging his parishioners not to go there. This ill will did their fledgling enterprise no good.

As before, they sought guidance in meditation. In this way, the idea came to them to revamp the facility to serve the many orphans in the area as a children's home and school; the clinic would continue, but it would be allotted a smaller space. Since Nigeria has many, many orphans, and only a few of the churches are able to care for them or educate them, the Omenkas figured this idea would meet with little resistance—and they were right.

The clinic, which once occupied five rooms, is now housed in one large room. Two of Ikechukwu's brothers, Martin and Chris, manage the clinic and are available to do treatments during day and evening hours. Volunteers from around the world also visit the clinic and offer their Reiki-charged hands in service. Additional permanent staff and volunteers run the Reiki Children's Home, which provides housing, food, and education for seventeen orphans of elementary and secondary school age. Although the children are not taught Reiki, staff may send distant healing to them if they contract malaria or another illness; Reiki is also used to help them calm down when they act out or get upset. The goal is to help the children recover from the emotional trauma of losing a parent or another family member to religious riots, tribal war, or illness.

Ikechukwu's dream is to bring the children of enemies together so that they will come to know and understand one another. "When we take children from the north, east, south, and west of Nigeria," he explains, "the big gift is that people bring in their own experience and *share*. They try to communicate . . . and then there will be a clear-washed human being. Now children restored to the family will be the ones to *end* the war, to say, 'forgive' and 'let's solve the problem.'" He hopes that when the children graduate from the school at the Reiki Children's Home and Clinic, they'll bring peace back to their homes and villages. Knowing that peace is possible, they can teach peace, too.

Although Ikechukwu's wife Ursula died in September 2006, he continues to be involved with the nonprofit foundation that guides the school and clinic, the Association for International Meeting Reiki-Nigeria. He remains the project manager and the contact person. For more information about volunteering or making a contribution to the Reiki Children's Home and Clinic, e-mail Ikechukwu Omenka at info@reiki-klinik-nigeria.com. The website www.reiki-klinik-nigeria.com provides some details about volunteer opportunities and offers many photos to provide a window to the world's first Reiki orphanage.

Be aware that Ikechukwu dreams big dreams. Recently, he returned to Nigeria to determine how to realize the next project. He would like to use the large plot of land he and his wife originally purchased to expand the home and school to house a thousand orphans. He would also like to staff the school with Montessori-trained teachers, who could address the individual learning needs of these traumatized children with the greatest sensitivity and care.

Ikechukwu set aside his own anger long ago. He has forgiven. What he and his family and friends have created is a miracle of healing in a land still struggling to emerge from war. Should you decide to visit and volunteer, be prepared for joy: the sudden, glorious realization that good can overcome, that forgiveness can mend broken families, and that peace is possible in a devastated country "just for today."

NOW YOU:
SEND REIKI HEALING FOR PEACE

We live on a planet that's under siege in many places, and in others it's recovering. While the war in Iraq continues and its resolution is unclear, the citizens of other countries, where other recent battles have been fought, clear away rubble and struggle to rebuild. How long does the process of recovery take? In our own country, recovery from the Civil War took generations and, in some pockets of the South, might be said to be still under way.

If recovery is such a long and arduous process, why does any nation go to war against another? Why do some countries suffer civil and tribal wars within their own borders? Political differences; racial and ethnic prejudice; religious intolerance; and greed over land and mineral rights, oil, and other natural resources are all used as excuses for making the first strike, aggressive action against another nation or faction within the same nation. This, of course, provides another excuse for war: defense and retaliation.

How can anyone resist being caught up in the fervor of a nation bent on war? First, remember that war is anathema to anyone who loves peace. The Dalai Lama now lives in exile in the West, lecturing and writing on peace, rather than in his homeland of Tibet, which was invaded by the Chinese in 1950 and remains occupied. Dr. Chujiro Hayashi, one of Mikao Usui's closest followers and Hawayo Takata's teacher, made his transition from this life in the spring of 1940 rather than face being called out of retirement to serve as an officer in the Japanese Navy during the Second World War. He was intent on living by the Reiki principles: "Just for today, do not anger" and "Be kind." Perhaps, inspired by the courage of such spiritual leaders, we may find ways to become stronger advocates of peace.

Second, come to know the "enemy," for knowledge has the power to overcome ignorance and intolerance. Learn to accept and appreciate differences in race, ethnic origin, religion, and cultural background; above all, recognize shared humanity. This "stranger" is your relative: another brother, sister, mother, father, or child in the human family. Be willing to set aside differences, share blessings, and offer kindness.

Finally, when you can, send Reiki healing for peace to the whole earth, or to the people and leaders of nations on the verge of war or already at war. If you're already trained to do Reiki distant healing, you can use the method you were taught. Simply change the wording of your intention in whatever way is appropriate to the situation; for example, "I offer Reiki healing for peace to _____ and _____ (name the countries involved) for the highest good of all concerned."

If you're trained to do hands-on Reiki only, you can still work with Reiki and your intention to send healing for peace. Simply raise your hands to heart level, hold them a few inches apart with your palms facing one another, and imagine or visualize the whole earth, or the geographic area at risk of war, between your palms. Feel the Reiki energy flow to the situation. Add your intention and any prayers for peace that seem appropriate. When your hands become quiet, say "thank you" in your heart and mind for this chance to send healing and for all healing that has occurred. Then bring your hands together, as if in prayer, to end the session, and go on with your normal activities. When you can, learn Reiki distant healing to add the power of the second level and the focus of the Reiki symbols to your practice.

There are many Reiki practitioners who daily send Reiki to the earth for healing and for peace. Some commit to this voluntary activity through an organization called Reiki Outreach International, established in 1990 by Mary McFadyen, a Reiki master trained by Hawayo Takata. That organization, now directed by Reiki Master Ann Thevenin, posts on its website suggested situations to address with Reiki distant healing and "instructions for transmission." The vision of the organization is to join tens of thousands of practitioners each day in sending Reiki healing ". . . towards famine, drought, plagues, mass illness, wars, political turmoil, and suffering of all kind[s] on the planet." To learn more, visit the Reiki Outreach International website at www.annieo.com/reikioutreach. Again, Reiki practitioners at all levels are welcome to join and participate in sending healing energy.

William Rand, of the International Center for Reiki Training, provides another resource for Reiki practitioners worldwide who wish to send Reiki for planetary healing and peace. He placed crystal grids at the North and South Poles in May 1997 and December 1999 respectively, and a third crystal grid in Jerusalem in October 2004. Each grid is intended to serve as a focal point for distant healing and is programmed to amplify Reiki in all directions. To see pictures of the World Peace Crystal Grids and learn more about them, visit the website at www.reiki.org/GlobalHealing/Northandsouthpolehomepage.html.

SUMMARY

The first principle, "Just for today, do not anger," challenges all Reiki practitioners to refuse to be provoked into antagonism by troublesome people or difficult circumstances. Fortunately, the quiet, steady flow of the energy through our hands is naturally tranquilizing. The more we practice hands-on and distant healing, the more familiar we become with the spiritual quality of peace. As we come to be more at peace with ourselves, it becomes easier to apply the first principle in our daily lives when we're confronted with argumentative people or frustrating situations.

As we continue to practice Reiki and recite the principles, we may become aware of present circumstances triggering anger that originated in the distant past. This, too, we are invited to heal by using the Reiki energy and by exploring the memories and emotions that arise, so that we can understand, forgive, and let go. While engaging in deliberate reflection and creative expression can help us confront our feelings in a safe setting, sometimes receiving counseling or participating in a support group can speed our emotional and mental healing even more.

Over time, as we see how effectively Reiki heals old anger and dissolves tension in our daily affairs, we may want to join in the effort of the global community of Reiki practitioners to bring peace to the world. We may use whatever Reiki distant-healing methods we've learned formally or a simplified method to send Reiki to the whole planet, to an area threatened by war, or to locations where war is already being fought. We may also request the energy flow to the leaders of nations for their highest guidance. In the aftermath of war or skirmishes, we can send Reiki to help the land recover and the people rebuild their lives.

MORE SUGGESTIONS FOR PRACTICE

❧ Did you ever become angry with someone with whom you couldn't communicate your feelings at all? Sometimes geographical distance puts us at this disadvantage; at other times social status or professional role makes it inappropriate for us to utter a single word of protest at the injustice or mistreatment we feel we've endured. What can we do with this justifiable anger, especially when the first Reiki principle recommends against being angry altogether? If we repress anger, pushing it down until it manifests as "issues in the tissues," we'll still probably have to explore these negative feelings thoroughly to free ourselves of them. What other options do we have?

Writing in a journal each day can be helpful and healing. We can use journals for many purposes, from keeping a chronological account of events to recording dreams, but if we vent our negative feelings on a blank page from time to time, then they'll be less likely to present themselves for our attention as the symptoms of physical stress or illness. While some people can use a journal for letting go of anger and anxiety on an "as needed" basis, most find that writing in a journal for a few minutes each day is more effective at keeping inner tension from building to dangerous levels. An added benefit of this practice is greater clarity of mind. As we express our feelings on the page, we find that confusion clears and our mood improves. We feel more competent and capable of solving the problems we face.

❧ Jungian psychologist Ira Progoff is responsible for developing journal-keeping into a genuinely therapeutic tool. He taught the Intensive Journal method to several thousand students during the last decades of the twentieth century. In his book, *At a Journal Workshop,* he describes many exercises for dialoguing with the body, the past, work projects, and other people. These exercises enable the writer to become more aware of negative feelings and let them go. To learn more about these techniques, visit your nearest bookstore and search the shelves. *At a Journal Workshop* is still in print and available for purchase as a new or used book.

❧ Another way to diffuse anger without harming anyone is to write a letter that you don't send. Use ordinary notebook paper and any pen or pencil on hand to say what you would really like to say face to face. As you do this, you may cry, scowl, smile, or laugh. As the words flow onto the page, feeling flows through you and you free yourself of them. You'll know when you've said all you need to say, because you'll feel lighter, as if the sun has shone within you and nothing hides in dark corners anymore. Your fears are gone. Your anger is expressed. Your hurt is healing—and acceptance of the situation is now possible. Do you send the letter? There's probably no need to do so. The letter has served its purpose, which is to bring you emotional release and closure, so that you can begin healing. You may want to put it away in a safe place, perhaps a locked drawer or a safe-deposit box, and look at it sometime in the future. Or you may want to burn the letter to symbolize that you're letting these feelings go.

❧ Yet another way to diffuse anger before it builds is to engage in "pillow talk." This is an exercise sometimes used by psychotherapists to help clients safely express their anger. Do you want to tell someone off? Grab a pillow, and let it sit in for your cranky boss, your difficult stepmother, or your temperamental teenager. Pretend. Say just what you want to say. Feel your feelings. Express them. Get them out of your body and into the air, where they'll do no harm. Feel like punching the jerk? Let the pillow have it and dissipate the force of your anger. This is an exercise that requires the privacy of a room with a closed door and enough time for you to process the feelings that are upsetting you. Again, you'll know when you've completed the exercise because you will feel better. As you feel yourself calming down, help your own healing along by doing some hands-on Reiki and getting some rest. Fighting—even with a pillow—can take a lot out of you.

❧ When we become angry, we give a lot of personal energy to an intense emotion. Sometimes the best way to diffuse the anger is not to direct that energy at anyone but to redirect it into a harmless activity that demands physical effort. Sweeping a kitchen floor is a time-honored way to burn off some of the heat of anger, but baking pies or swinging a hammer can also work well. One day, when I found myself unable to walk off a "mad," an empty plastic bag blew right into my path; I realized that I could adopt the road for the next hour or so and pick up every recyclable item I saw on the shoulder. Do you have an activity or chore on your to-do list that demands enough physical effort to make it a good way to diffuse anger? The next time you feel tempted to turn on someone or yourself in fury, remind yourself that this task needs to be done and do it. Build, bake, or create something beautiful—and burn off the personal energy you put into anger in a positive way.

❧ Laughter can lighten tension in some situations, diffusing anger the way a pinprick deflates a balloon. While it is not always appropriate to laugh when you are being confronted or challenged, sometimes it works to shift energy in a positive way. Even when it is not appropriate at the time, reflecting on the situation later and discovering the humor in it "lets off some steam." You can look for the laughter on your own, thinking back on the incident or writing about it in a journal. You can also talk to a friend and transform remembered tension into an excuse for camaraderie. If you think you need help in understanding how to see the funny side of your own situation, spend some time listening to comedians, live and on stage, or on TV or DVD. Their material is often drawn from ordinary life and its difficulties. They demonstrate the many ways to see the humor in personal disaster. Learn from them.

❧ Do you know where you hold anger in your body? If you like to draw, have a go at an informal self-portrait. Use shelf paper or newsprint and crayons that won't allow precision. Quickly sketch the shape of your head, neck, shoulders, torso, arms, and legs. Now close your eyes and notice where you hold tension in your body. Give that tension a color and find it in the crayon box. Draw it onto your self-portrait. Close your eyes again. Let yourself become more aware of your physical body. Whenever you feel tension, stress, upset, or ache, pick a color and draw a bit more. When your drawing feels complete, have a good look. Can you tell what situations in your life are causing the tension in each area? This exercise can bring up feelings that have been suppressed for days, weeks, and even years. Allow yourself adequate time to process the feelings that arise, understand them, and let them go. This provides some closure. Doing this exercise with a partner, who can listen to you express the feelings that arise without judgment can also serve this need. For help, you may want to turn to Louise Hay's book, *You Can Heal Your Life,* and for inspiration see the movie of the same name, released in 2008. If her correlations of mind and body make sense to you, consider using the affirmations she offers for your healing, or create a few affirmations of your own.

❧ As you attempt to live by the Reiki principles in your daily life, make note of the anger management tools and techniques that work for you. Knowing you have these resources on call for coping with difficult emotions can provide an immediate sense of relief: this self-knowledge empowers you with an awareness of choice. You do not have to be overcome by anger. "Just for today," you *can* choose to be at peace.

4

SERENITY

"Just for Today, Do Not Worry"

Translators of the Reiki principles are in general accord about the English wording of the second principle: "Just for today, do not worry." Right now, do not be anxious; do not be concerned. Let your mind become quiet and calm. With peace of mind, whatever challenges you face will be easier to comprehend, understand, accept, and resolve. Focus on the present moment with relaxed awareness. See it in its simplicity as well as its complexity. Be aware that it holds opportunities and blessings, as well as unresolved problems and issues. Be grateful for those opportunities and blessings. Allow the light of your own consciousness to shine forth and show you the way that is open to you. Perhaps it won't be the way that you desired or expected. Still it's a way forward. Take it and be at peace, knowing that—just for today, just for now—you're doing the best you can.

When Reiki Master Beth Gray presented the Reiki principles to her students, she added one word of advice after "just for today, do not worry": "accept." This recommendation has great merit; when we're willing to calm our fears and accept the "reality" of our situation, we may also begin to understand how to create positive change. If we allow anxiety to escalate, then we may find ourselves feeling overwhelmed, depressed, paralyzed, and unable to take any effective action. Yet we have a choice: we can choose to focus our attention on something other than our worries. We can quiet our thoughts. We can look at the circumstances of our lives with mental clarity, emotional calm, and spiritual wisdom. In this way, we become more open and able to accept healing, through Reiki and other methods and means, both familiar and new to us.

REIKI TEACHES SERENITY

Reiki teaches us peace and acceptance. We can apply our hands to ease pain and to bring comfort. We can listen to the energy. We can do our best—and no more. If there are to be miracles, the energy will accomplish them. If there is to be remarkable healing, the energy will bring it forth. If there is to be only minor healing, the energy will bring this about as well. We're not in charge of the outcome. We do our best and hope for the best, and in the process, we gradually learn to trust the energy and to better understand its nature. Takata called Reiki "God-power"; Beth Gray called Reiki "the energy of unconditional love." The recommendation, "Just for today, do not worry," invites us to extend our trust to the Source of universal life-force energy, and in doing so, to claim more than mere acceptance. We are beckoned forward on our spiritual path to a place where we may consider faith and even something beyond faith: serenity, the knowledge that we are intimately known, deeply loved, and always guided by Spirit.

IN THE FACE OF CHANGE

Although we live in a world where disaster sometimes strikes on a global scale, decimating the populations of small nations or destroying the coastline of half a continent, most of us don't face disaster on a daily basis. We face smaller "worries," such as the threat of unemployment; the fear of loneliness; difficulties in communication with a family member; a nagging, undiagnosed medical problem; a shortfall of cash at the end of the month; or concern over how best to care for an aging relative. Inevitably though, our sense of security is threatened not only by the possibility of negative change but also by the prospect of positive change: starting an exciting, new job; accepting a long-awaited marriage proposal; moving to a different city; having a baby; adopting a pet; joining a sports team; being asked to sing a solo in a choir; finding a great apartment; buying a house; renting out a room to a tenant; or welcoming a widowed parent into our home.

What makes our lives so full, rich, and "interesting" is that often we must cope with multiple, stressful changes at the same time, both positive and negative; and most positive changes are rarely unalloyed. For example, marriage to a wonderful partner might bring with it the problem of acceptance by three difficult teenage stepchildren. A move to a new city and higher paying job may require giving up a beloved house in a country setting. Accepting a terrific promotion might come with the responsibility for firing some of our coworkers.

Every day brings changes, and some changes are difficult to accept. The ability to welcome change, embrace it, and adapt to it is resilience. We're all born with some degree of natural resilience, and we can learn to cultivate it as well. If not, if we resist change and fail to adapt to it, then we risk suffering physical and emotional consequences, such as tension headaches, stiff necks, aching lower backs, indigestion, heartburn, insomnia, anxiety attacks, depression, and more. We ignore such symptoms at our own peril. Prolonged periods of extreme stress compromise immunity, making us more susceptible to infections of all kinds, and increase the risk of heart disease, cancer, and other life-threatening medical conditions.

Fortunately, Reiki offers a healthy way to relax in response to the challenges we face in our lives. Simple hands-on Reiki healing can help dissolve the physical tension in someone whose day at the office was so bad that it evoked the fight-or-flight response and sent adrenaline levels soaring. Reiki can calm the racing heart of a person experiencing a panic attack after witnessing a shooting. It can quiet the sobs of someone at a funeral who feels overwhelmed by grief. It can ease a mental stranglehold, when we're unable to face or sort out problems, for it quiets the emotions and clears the mind. In other words, Reiki can help us feel more resilient, more relaxed about whatever challenges we face, clearer-headed, calmer, and better able to cope.

Like all people, Reiki practitioners have choices about how to respond to sudden crises, isolated or repeated anxiety-provoking events, and the "daily grind"—the relentless, tension-inducing routine of early-morning rush-hour traffic; tedium behind a desk; touch-and-go attempts to make it out of work on time; and a frenzied rush home. We may express or repress our feelings. We may attend to problems as they arise and attempt to resolve them or avoid or deny their existence. We may choose to be fully present to our experience in each moment and able to avail ourselves of all our inner and external resources or we may allow our attention to be diverted from the present by instead responding with a behavior pattern learned in the past, such as caretaking, mediating, acting out, blame casting, overachieving, underachieving, aiming for mediocrity to avoid attention, or escaping into alcohol or drugs.

Reiki practitioners, however, may make another choice: to practice Reiki and attempt to live by the Reiki principles. We can use Reiki on ourselves to alleviate our own anxiety and tension; send Reiki healing to any current or future situations that concern us so that they will resolve in whatever way is for the highest good; and send Reiki healing to any past events that left us traumatized, anxious, or feeling unable to cope. We can recite the Reiki principles morning and night, affirming our intention to live by the values they express; we can be mindful of them throughout the day; and when confronted with an unwelcome challenge or change, we can breathe through the moment of crisis, silently repeating, "Just for today, do not worry."

THE ANSWER TO MRS. TAKATA'S PRAYERS

Most Reiki practitioners and teachers don't know much about Hawayo Takata's early life, instead focusing on the incredible contributions she made once she learned Reiki; for example, setting up the first Reiki treatment center in the Western hemisphere, in her home state of Hawaii; teaching countless people to do Reiki hands-on and distant healing; and finally, in the mid-1970s, training twenty-two Reiki masters, who traveled widely establishing Reiki around the world. She taught Reiki with great love and deep integrity, with respect for her teacher and for the Reiki energy as teacher, and she appreciated both the lessons of her life and its many blessings.

Did she ever face difficulties that caused her to worry? Yes. Before learning Reiki, the young Hawayo Takata, wife and mother of two small children, lost her husband Saichi Takata to lung cancer. During the next five years, she struggled to support her family. In *Living Reiki: Takata's Teachings,* Fran Brown writes:

> She worked very hard to become financially able to care for her family. She had little rest, pushing herself to hide her grief, to the point where she had a nervous breakdown. She also had a painful abdominal condition, a uterine tumor, which required surgery, and emphysema from asthma, which prevented the use of an anesthetic.[1]

Takata had quite a lot to worry about! Yet in the five years after her husband's death, she developed the habit of sitting under a camphor tree to rest and to "meditate and pray." One day, feeling particularly low, she pleaded with God to hear her prayers—and then she heard an inner voice: "Yes, you have many troubles. Listen well . . . the first thing is to take care of your health and that of your family. If you have good health, you shall have wealth, because you can work and you can earn. You shall have happiness, security, and long life."[2] Takata felt profound gratitude to have received such an answer. Yet she continued to pray for guidance, for she didn't know how to begin following this advice and reclaiming her health.

Three weeks later, one of Takata's sisters died suddenly. This was such sad news that she felt she must deliver it in person to her parents, who had retired to Japan. So she readied herself for the trip, planning to visit her parents, return her husband's ashes to his homeland, and visit the Maeda Clinic for her own health treatment. When she arrived in Japan, she was admitted as a patient at the Maeda Clinic, diagnosed, and scheduled for immediate surgery.

Yet once more, she heard an inner voice, which prompted her to ask the doctors and nurses preparing for the operation whether there was an alternative. On the basis of the chief surgeon's information about Dr. Chujiro Hayashi's clinic, Takata refused the operation. Instead, she went to Hayashi's clinic where she was treated with Reiki over many months. This allowed her to recover her health and to focus on a new purpose in life: to offer Reiki healing to others at home in Hawaii, and later, to teach Reiki healing in Hawaii and wherever she was invited throughout the United States and Canada.

Because of Takata's willingness to meditate and pray, she was open to hearing inner guidance. Because she felt unclear, she prayed for further guidance. As the events of her life unfolded, she followed the direction she was shown to reclaim her health. She received additional inner guidance just as conventional surgery was to take place, and this "course correction" set her feet firmly on the path to Reiki.

HOPING FOR MIRACLES

Iryna Zhyrenko, whose journey to Reiki began in Russia with hope forged out of grief over her father's death, arrived in the United States determined to learn more about Reiki and pursue her training to the master level. When she contacted me in the fall of 2001 and explained her interest, I was happy to talk to her and intrigued by the story she told. When I described how I teach Reiki master students, requiring them to attend four full weekends of instruction and assist at three level I and three level II classes over the course of nine to twelve months, she was not put off by the stringency of the requirements or the time commitment she would have to make. Instead, she was enthusiastic about finding a teacher who wanted to support students in integrating the experience of the master attunement and to prepare them with the knowledge and the teaching skills they would need to feel confident in the classroom.

Iryna's only worry was how to pay for Reiki master training. She felt good about her decision to take a comprehensive training program in teaching traditional Reiki. Yet she still had to find a way to come up with the money to pay for the course. She didn't know what to do. She didn't feel comfortable asking her new husband for the money, so she decided to do some meditation and ask for God's help in prayer. At some point during the meditation, she fell asleep.

Iryna was awakened by the sound of a ringing phone. Someone who had seen her advertisement in the Russian community paper was calling to ask to see one of the beautiful, purebred ragdoll kittens that recently had been born to her cat, Minnie. Despite the fact that the ad had run for several weeks, this was the first inquiry Iryna had received. The caller visited her later that night and bought one of the kittens for $650. The next day, Iryna received another phone call from someone who wanted to buy a purebred ragdoll kitten. This visit, too, resulted in the sale of a kitten and several hundred dollars more in Iryna's bank account. She called to tell me of her Reiki miracle and to assure me that she would be a member of the Reiki master class scheduled to start soon. So, with just a little meditation and prayer, Iryna's money worries went away. It became possible for her to pursue a dream that had begun in Russia two years before, in the dark, lonely days after her father's death, when she had wondered how to heal her grief and rebuild her life.

THE POWER OF
MEDITATION AND PRAYER

For the young, widowed Mrs. Takata, overwrought with worries about her own health and her family's welfare, meditation and prayer brought comfort—and the spiritual guidance she needed to move forward with her life. In Takata's story of Mikao Usui's life, Usui turned to meditation and prayer for guidance on whether to bring this ancient healing method, lost for so long, back into the world, and he turned to it again to come to an understanding of where to begin his healing work. His meditation, prayer vigil, and fast on Mt. Kurama ended with his spontaneous attunement to Reiki and his empowerment to bring about great healing. Entering into meditation and prayer is a time-honored way to seek inner peace and guidance.

NOW YOU: DISCOVER REIKI AS
HEALING MEDITATION

There are many ways to meditate. Most meditation techniques direct the practitioner to focus the mind on a particular point, process, or sound. For example, one simple way to meditate is to look upon the flickering light of a candle flame. Study the flame, then close your eyes, and see if you can visualize the flame and hold the image. When the image becomes unstable, look at the candle flame again. Another technique is to focus on following your breath, gently bringing your attention back to the sensations of inhalation or exhalation any time that your mind strays. Another common practice is to use a mantra, a sacred word or sound that you simply repeat, sometimes chanting it out loud again and again, sometimes chanting it silently. This method, too, brings the mind's attention to a task, so awareness becomes more focused, emotions become calm, and the body becomes more relaxed.

Meditation can also mean deliberate contemplation of an idea, such as eternity, love, or the nature of the Divine. Such meditations become ongoing reflections and affect the practitioner's mind in the same way that a stone dropped into a still pond sends out rippling waves. This book invites meditation on the Reiki principles in that way and also in the way that Mikao Usui recommended: mindful chanting, morning and night.

Even much less formal meditations can have powerfully healing effects, because whenever we remove our attention from our worries and concerns and focus it instead on something soothing or comforting, we rest and heal. In these few moments of diversion, we also allow our subconscious minds time and space to solve problems, so that when we reconsider the worrisome situation, we discover that we're refreshed; now we can think of solutions that hadn't occurred to us before. Sitting by a window and watching—really watching—birds at a bird feeder can divert us in this way. A walk along a country road or an easy hike on a mountain path can connect us to nature and the rhythm of our breathing to relax worry's hold. Knitting, sketching, and working a jigsaw puzzle can all rest the frustrated and weary conscious mind, so the childlike subconscious can later play magician, offering up creative new solutions to us as if pulling rabbits out of a hat.

Doing Reiki, too, can be a meditation. Whether we're distracted or preoccupied as we start a hands-on treatment, we discover that our minds quickly become quiet and calm as we focus on the flow of Reiki energy. Although we may first notice the energy as it radiates through our hands, as we give it more attention, we may become aware of it entering through the crown and flowing down along the spinal column, and then through our arms and hands. In this simple way, we become centered. We may even discover that when we close our eyes, we see a beautiful swirl of color or a wash of sparkling light. As we enjoy watching this inner show, the energy brings us more healing. Gradually, we come to realize that in the peace of Reiki, we're brought to a gentle awareness of our own connection to Source.

When we enter this altered state, we are more mindful of the healing presence of Spirit. We experience peace. We may also experience other qualities that are associated with Spirit: unconditional love, compassion, benevolence, kindness, comfort, and guidance. This guidance, which may come to us in the form of an image, a voice, or a "knowing" without knowing how we know, may bring encouragement, reassurance, direction, or the answer to a prayer.

Please understand that, when doing Reiki in the traditional way, there's no requirement to pay attention to anything but the resonance of the energy in your hands so that you'll know when to shift them to another position; and once learned, this ability becomes automatic, something you can easily do while conversing, reading a book, or watching a movie. Letting your mind wander, reviewing your day's to-do list, or rehearsing your lines for a speech as your hands transfer healing energy is absolutely fine—and sometimes quite necessary. Deliberate thought about something else or simple distraction does not lessen the flow of Reiki through your hands or reduce the quantity or quality of healing that your client receives. This is true even when you're treating yourself. *You* are not doing the healing, so where you put your mind's attention will not affect the flow of Reiki. Reiki is the healer, and Reiki, or universal life-force energy, taps an infinite well.

At times, however, you will find that you have the opportunity to be mindful as you do Reiki. You may give your complete attention to the sensations you feel in your hands. Or, as you continue to practice over time and develop increasingly subtle perception, you may choose to divide your attention between your hands and the flow of the energy as it enters through the crown of your head and travels downward through your body. Eventually, this won't seem like "dividing" your attention at all, because you'll be aware of yourself as being at one with the energy. Relax into the flow of Reiki, appreciate how it gently brings you healing, and allow yourself to accept the gift. Sometimes, when the energy comes in waves, you can even breathe in rhythm with it. If you liked body surfing in the ocean as a child, this is an experience you'll definitely enjoy.

If you are intent upon experiencing Reiki as meditation, schedule an appointment with yourself. Choose a time when you will be awake, alert, and unlikely to be interrupted so that you can give your relaxed attention to the subtle sensations of energy in and around your hands. Then be fully present to your experience. Perhaps you notice warmth in your heart or tingling in your feet as the energy flows through your physical body and energy field. Good. Just notice and appreciate your experience. If you find your mind drifting away to a worry or concern, tell yourself that you'll deal with that issue later and let it go. Gently bring your attention back to the flow of the energy.

When you are treating a scheduled client, you may also have the opportunity to be mindful. Honor the client's request for background music or silence and then give yourself up to the experience of the Reiki energy. Sense it as fully as you can, without either expectation or demand. Do you feel just a mild hum of current in your hands? Good. Do you feel so merged with the energy that your hands seem to have disappeared? Good. Be willing to be with the energy as you do Reiki, whether the sensations you experience are mild or intense, and whether they seem simple or multidimensional. Make the choice to be fully present to the experience of your own healing. Being mindful of the energy's flow is a way to honor the presence of Spirit; it is also a way to be open to guidance.

PRAYER:
SURRENDERING YOUR WORRIES

Ellen Phillips, who co-teaches a workshop on the Reiki principles with me, sometimes tells this story to our students: one day, she was driving her little red Volkswagen hatchback on a narrow, winding country road near her house. As usual, she felt intense anxiety about being in a car. Whether behind the wheel or in the passenger's seat, she had never felt very safe. Because of this, she had avoided making long car trips for most of her life. Now a friend had offered her the opportunity to be hypnotized to cure her phobia. *Why do I have to be hypnotized?* she wondered. *Why can't I just ask Dr. Usui for help in healing this phobia and have it go away?* This was not an idle question: Ellen is trained to use the second Reiki symbol not only for mental and emotional healing but also for intuitive communication;* she often asks Mikao Usui for guidance in her life. And so, in the silence of her mind, she asked him for help with her phobia as she continued driving with her eyes on the road. Immediately, she felt all her anxiety dissolve and a remarkable sense of peace descend upon her. Ever since this experience, she has felt completely at ease when traveling by car.

Here is a story that I sometimes share in the same workshop: one night, just before I drifted off to sleep, I said a quick prayer, closed my eyes, and surrendered to sleep. Perhaps twenty minutes later, I was awakened by a sudden popping sound and a flash of light, and then another in quick succession at the side of the bed nearest the wall. I looked down and saw more sparks flying around the electrical outlet. With my heart pounding, I realized that there was a burning smell in the air. I hurried to find a flashlight, turned it on, and shone it at the outlet and the mattress to see if the sparks had become flames. No. I let out a long breath. On the way out of my room, I glanced at my alarm clock, which normally glows red at night; I saw only a dull black face. I flicked the light switch by the door, but nothing happened. The near-fire had flipped the circuit breaker in the basement. Once that was remedied, I turned the light on in the room and discovered the cause of the problem: an electrical cord had been too close to the baseboard radiator and had melted and then sparked. I remembered my brief prayer and thanked the angels for watching over me.

NOW YOU:
DISCOVER THE POWER OF PRAYER

As Reiki practitioners, we are profoundly connected to Source or Spirit. When we are attuned, the natural ability that we have to bring healing to one another through touch is greatly enhanced; it's expanded, stabilized, reinforced, and sealed from negativity. We become conscious channels of

---

*For more about this technique, please see my book *Intuitive Reiki for Our Times: Essential Techniques for Enhancing Your Practice*.

universal life-force energy. Whether or not we're religious, as we practice over time, we begin to realize that the healing energy that flows through our hands is delivered by a higher power. One of our spiritual lessons is learning to trust that power.

If we were raised to practice a particular religion, we may discover that our experience of Reiki fits perfectly into our existing understanding of the nature of God. We may find that our faith seems renewed. We may enjoy prayer more, for we have more evidence in our lives that prayers are answered. If we were brought up as agnostics or atheists, we may find that our worldview gradually shifts and becomes more accommodating of the idea of a higher power. Prayer does not feel comfortable or natural to us at all. Yet we may find ourselves asking whatever is the source of the Reiki energy for help in healing a particular friend, family member, or situation, and when we do, we're on the way to praying.

"Spirit, help me with this, please." Prayer can be that simple. Reiki practitioners who are members of a church, meeting, synagogue, mosque, or temple will be familiar with prayers of their faith. Those who were brought up without learning traditional prayers may feel more comfortable seeking help from the Reiki "guides," especially Mikao Usui, or their guardian angels. Although we're all surely protected, loved, and guided by Spirit throughout our lives, certain help is available to us only if we ask. So why not ask? Why not experiment with prayer and see what happens?

Yes, we have the Reiki energy and the Reiki symbols. We may beam Reiki around the bedroom where we'll soon fall asleep. We may visualize the symbols, especially the first symbol, on the steering wheel of our car before we drive off or all around the hull of an airplane before we fly to our destination. There is tremendous protective power in both actions. Perhaps, we might also enjoy the help of angels. There's only one way to find out: pray. Test out old, familiar prayers. Make up prayers in your own words. Mikao Usui meditated and prayed on Mt. Kurama. Hawayo Takata meditated and prayed under the camphor tree. Focus your awareness on the higher power that guides the healing energy that flows through your hands and set down your worries. Ask for the help you need. Pray.

REIKI FOR STRESS AT WORK

Lauren Sage (mentioned in chapter 1) is a wife and mother who holds an MBA; she is also a Reiki master. She heads a department of fifty people in the corporate offices of a large pharmaceutical manufacturer. Each fall, she and her department are called upon to write a section of the company's annual report that requires many hours of data input and statistical analysis. Typically, Lauren puts in fifteen-hour days and works seven days a week for about three months, managing her staff, overseeing the project, and writing large sections of the report.

Yet out of long habit, every morning before she even gets out of bed, Lauren does Reiki on herself. She often finds that in the very first position, over the lower rib cage, the Reiki flow is intense as the energy sinks through her body to strengthen her adrenal glands, which can get depleted during extreme on-the-job stress.

As she does Reiki, Lauren recalls the Reiki principles. She lets the words, "Just for today, do not worry," fill her mind. Then she thinks about the day's meetings, staff management problems, and project deadlines—and lets her worries about them go. She visualizes everything coming together easily and anticipates everything working out well. "Even though I'm under a lot of pressure and I'm not getting a lot of sleep," she says, "I haven't felt exhausted or gotten sick. I feel fine. I think the Reiki energy really keeps my immune system strong—and reminding myself, 'Just for today, do not worry' really helps."

NOW YOU:
USE REIKI TO IMPROVE YOUR WORK

Whenever you can, before you go to work, begin your day with a recitation of the Reiki principles and with Reiki self-treatment. If you are an advanced practitioner and you have moments to spare, send Reiki forward in time to be received as needed throughout the day; you may also want to send Reiki to any long-term or large, complex work projects to speed their successful completion.

Think of Mikao Usui climbing Mt. Kurama, knowing that when he arrived at the top, he would begin a twenty-one-day meditation and fast. Did he worry as he walked up the mountain? He had a clear purpose, and he had made a commitment to Spirit. It seems more likely that before he began he set all worries aside. He knew what he must do, he set out to do it, and he did it.

Imagine that you are able to approach your work in the same way: be clear-minded, decisive, and calm. Be committed to your spiritual practice. Do what you know to do next, without becoming emotional about it. Be mindful of the Reiki principles throughout the day, especially "Just for today, do not worry." You may find that you are enjoying your work life more than you ever thought possible.

REIKI TO COPE WITH A DEMANDING SCHEDULE

Lauren Bissett (introduced in the first chapter), who came to Reiki as a burn patient, recently graduated from community college with her associate's degree and her certification as a registered nurse in hand. In addition to her classroom studies, she worked eight to twelve hour shifts during the week at various local hospitals doing her clinical internship. Like many full-time community-college students, Lauren also worked part time as a waitress to pay her rent and her way through school.

Although she's young and healthy, and was highly motivated to achieve her goal of becoming a nurse specializing in burn care, Lauren found that she had to squeeze in study time late at night. This often left her tired the next day. By the end of the semester, she felt run down. To cope with this demanding schedule, she did hands-on and distant Reiki healing on herself whenever she could. When she sensed a tension headache building up from fatigue or felt jittery before a test, she did hado breathing (introduced briefly in chapter 1), a technique presented by Hiroshi Doi in his workshops on Usui Reiki Ryoho (traditional Japanese Reiki) and Gendai (modern) Reiki during his numerous visits to the West.[3]

Here's how to do hado breathing:

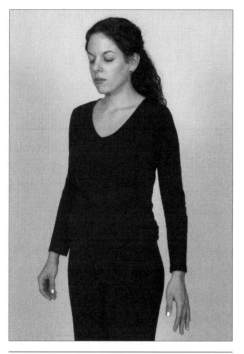

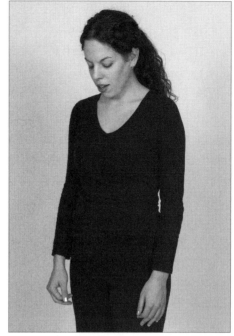

Figure 4.1   Figure 4.2

1. As you sit or stand in a comfortable posture, take a slow, deep breath, filling your lungs and letting your chest and shoulders lift (fig. 4.1). Hold the breath until you feel the impulse to exhale.
2. Now exhale, forcibly expelling all the air in your lungs and making any sound that seems appropriate to you. As you do, let your shoulder muscles sag downward as you relax all physical tension (fig. 4.2). (Most practitioners heave a big, noisy sigh when they try this breathing technique. Lauren says that the sound she usually makes is more like a growl than a sigh, so she's careful to practice hado breathing in the privacy of her car or apartment.)

By using hands-on Reiki and this technique, Lauren found that she was able to cope with her workload most days without complaint. However, when she felt particularly overwhelmed or faced a test in one of her courses, she asked for help. By phone or e-mail, she requested that her name be placed on a Reiki distant-healing list sent to many practitioners. Once she did that, she relaxed and trusted in the power of Reiki to bring healing on all levels.

How successful was she in coping with the stress of this strenuous schedule? "I did really well at school," she says. "Whenever I asked for Reiki to be sent to me forward in time when I knew I would be taking a test, I got high marks. It happened again and again!"

This spring, even before her graduation, Lauren was hired to work in the emergency room of a local hospital. By the time this book is published, she will have completed her Reiki master training and be certified to teach Reiki.

NOW YOU:
SEND REIKI FORWARD
IN TIME TO ANY SITUATION

In Reiki II, when practitioners learn a method of doing Reiki distant healing, they are always taught that it can be used to bring healing to clients in need, no matter how physically far away they are. Geographic distance doesn't matter. For example, a Reiki II practitioner in Arkansas can send healing to an aunt who has suffered a heart attack in Texas, a Reiki master might send Reiki to a student whose car has broken down on the way to class, or a group of Reiki practitioners at a Reikishare might gather in a circle to send Reiki to people suffering from famine in Africa. (Reikishares will be explained in more detail in chapter 7.)

What is not always taught is the versatility of Reiki distant healing. Not only can it be sent to a single client but also to a couple, a family, or a group; not only can it be sent to a person or group of people but also to a pet, farm animal, wild animal, or whole species. Not only can it be sent for physical, mental, or emotional healing but also to heal a situation or help achieve a goal. Not only can it be sent across geographic miles but also across time.

One of the simplest ways to use Reiki to alleviate worry over an event that hasn't yet occurred is to send distant healing forward in time to the situation, whether it's a dentist's appointment or major surgery, a meeting with a business client, or the hour of a friend's passing. To do this, use whatever distant healing method you habitually use, making a slight modification in the wording of intention.

Here's an example of the wording a practitioner might use before sending Reiki to a friend named Benjamin Miller, who's scheduled to have a tooth extraction during the coming week: "Benjamin Miller, Benjamin Miller, Benjamin Miller, I offer Reiki healing to you forward in time to be received as needed during your dental surgery on the afternoon of Tuesday, January 27. You are free to accept or reject this healing for your highest good and the highest good of all concerned." Here's another example, using a student's test-taking situation: "Miranda Jones, Miranda Jones, Miranda Jones, I offer you Reiki healing to be received as needed while you are taking your final exam in introductory psychology next week. You are free to accept or reject this healing for your highest good and the highest good of all concerned."

While there are many different methods and wordings of intention that may be used when doing Reiki distant healing, the statements above are specific and clear in naming the client and the future situation in need of healing, they indicate that the Reiki healing is an offering only and acknowledge that the client has free will to accept or refuse, and they release the outcome "for the highest good." This is important. It acknowledges that the Reiki practitioner is not in control of the outcome, nor is he or she attempting to manipulate results for personal ends. Miranda Jones will get an A on her final with the Reiki energy's help only if getting that A is in alignment with her soul's purpose and for her highest good.

There is a joy in the moment of surrendering the outcome to the energy, in releasing the future result to the wisdom of the higher power that guides all healing. Often, after we have done so, we're surprised by how much the universe supports us in bringing healing or achieving our goals. When the outcome is different from what we had hoped, we have the opportunity to practice another kind of surrender: acceptance of the wisdom of that higher power. This acceptance, too, is something we learn along the path of Reiki.

A SON IN PRISON:
REIKI AND COMMUNITY SUPPORT

Since Judi Taylor was widowed seven years ago, she has come to appreciate her son Caiden's inner strength, resilience, and courage. She has watched him grow out of boyhood without a father into a man who would make his father proud. She is certainly proud of Caiden for his dedication to his studies, his good manners, and his gentle nature and sensitivity to the needs of others.

So it was tremendously upsetting to her when Caiden, on fall break from his freshman year at college, was arrested as an accessory to a nightmarish crime that he did nothing to stop. A new acquaintance and his girlfriend invited Caiden to go out trick-or-treating with them on Halloween. Unknown to him, she carried a knife hidden in the folds of her costume. In the chilly autumn twilight, she stopped two young children who were passing by, and then pulled a knife and demanded the older child's haul of candy. Caiden looked on, shocked into stunned silence. The younger child immediately ran away, unharmed, but the older child stayed to protest, then left with the candy, frightened, but otherwise unharmed. However, Caiden and his two new acquaintances were charged with assault with a deadly weapon, which is a felony. At the preliminary hearing, the public defender convinced both boys to plead not guilty and go to trial. The judge reduced the charges against the girl because she was underage; he regarded her behavior as a juvenile prank. Caiden, who was twenty, would have to stand trial as an adult. Despite the prosecutor's request that he be given a two-year sentence, the judge took into account Caiden's unblemished record, good grades at school, and character. For his role as an accessory, he was sentenced to three months on work release in the county prison.

Nothing in Judi's life, except perhaps the death of her husband, had prepared her for the sense of loss and helplessness she felt when her son was admitted into the prison system. She was not even allowed to accompany him to the prison door. For the first few weeks of Caiden's sentence, while his paperwork was being processed and he waited to be assigned to group living quarters and a job, Judi wasn't allowed any contact with him, nor was he allowed to receive mail or any phone calls. Without this connection, Judi felt as if her own life was on hold, as all of her mental and emotional energy spiraled into a storm of fears around her son.

Of course, she sent Reiki to Caiden every day, and she did Reiki on herself as well. However, she believes that what made this difficult time bearable for her was reaching out to her spiritual community, which included many

Reiki practitioners. When she described Caiden's circumstances, she was met with sympathy, compassion, and understanding. She discovered that she wasn't alone in experiencing someone she loved "doing time." Someone even came forward who had served a sentence in the same prison to give her a sense of what Caiden's life would be like for the three months he would be there.

Judi asked for herself and her son to be placed on the Reiki distant-healing list from a few days after the charges were made through the hearing, the trial, and the months of his imprisonment. When he was released, she wrote a long e-mail to all those who had sent healing and prayers, thanking them for their support and acknowledging the lessons she and Caiden had learned about love, courage, and friendship, and the spiritual growth they had both experienced during that difficult time. By using Reiki on herself, sending it to her son Caiden, and asking for the support of other practitioners who sent Reiki to the situation, she found that she and her son could both endure the unthinkable and emerge stronger and wiser for it.

Judi also looked for the spiritual lessons hidden in this life-changing event. She was forced to let all her high hopes for Caiden's college future go—for now. She also discovered that she had no energy to put into playing the role of victim. If anyone had been treated unfairly, it was Caiden, but there was absolutely nothing to be gained by complaining to him, to God, or to anyone else that his sentence was unjust or life was so unfair. To support him, she herself would have to be strong, accepting the situation and acting with as much wisdom, grace, and dignity as she could muster. As she learned to live "just for today," letting go of worry, she realized that she had no choice but to trust Spirit to watch over Caiden, as, ultimately, every mother must do for every child.

This acceptance of the situation and trust in Spirit helped restore her peace of mind. With this perspective, she could see clearly which actions were appropriate for her to take to support her son during his prison sentence. She did what she could, asked for spiritual help and community support, and accepted what she could not do. This freed her to begin to focus more on her own life, reclaiming old interests and discovering new ones, a task that she had begun to engage in when Caiden entered college. By the time he was released, he had gained a greater sense of himself and his own strengths, and Judi knew and liked herself better as well. Mother and son had both "grown up"—and become much more independent and self-reliant. Separated by circumstances but united by love, they had turned personal tragedy into triumph.

NOW YOU:
ACCEPT THE SITUATION
AND TRUST SOURCE

A child leaves the nest to enter college, serve in the military, move to the city, backpack through Europe, hitchhike across country, join the Peace Corps, save the Amazon rainforest, or work on an oil rig in the Gulf of Mexico. A spouse leaves and never returns due to a fatal car accident. A spouse leaves with a good-bye kiss, as if setting off to work in the morning, but doesn't come home; instead, a letter from a lawyer and divorce papers arrive in the mail. A spouse leaves slowly, agonizingly, as Alzheimer's disease destroys memory and identity. A spouse dies peacefully of old age, while sleeping in bed at home. A parent suffers a fatal heart attack while shoveling heavy, wet snow. A sibling falls through thin ice while skating. A best friend moves to another state.

Life changes, and we do lose people, pets, houses, and jobs we love. Sometimes we're fortunate enough to have them restored to us for an hour, a few days, or a lifetime. Often, we are not. We must simply feel and express our grief, let go of the pain of loss, and then go on. We can be kind to ourselves when such events occur by allowing ourselves time and quiet solitude to heal and reflect. We may find that meditation and prayer become more important to us, bringing comfort, guidance, and a stronger sense of connection to Spirit. We may discover that writing in a journal or another form of creative expression is also a powerful healing tool, helping us set down the burden of emotional turmoil.

Reiki practitioners are fortunate to have additional resources: Reiki-charged hands to bring healing and the Reiki principles to invite reflection and guide each day's decisions. During this interlude, this interruption of ordinary life, we can give ourselves Reiki hands-on healing morning and

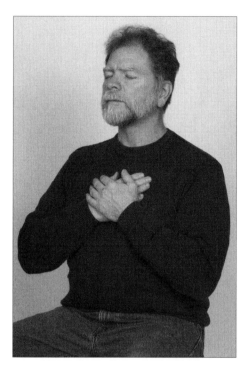

Daily self-treatment can help us cope in crises.

night, and send ourselves Reiki distant healing using a proxy or crystal grid all day long. We can ask for other Reiki practitioners to support us by sending us Reiki when they can, and ask for Reiki distant healing to be sent back in time to the moment of loss to help us recover and move forward. We can remind ourselves not to worry, and we can look for the blessings of each moment to bring ourselves back to now and back into an attitude of gratitude. This intense work on ourselves with Reiki will accelerate our healing on all levels.

As soon as we can accept the changed situation and come to terms with the loss, we'll begin to be able to see the landscape of our lives more clearly and decide when and how to move forward. This isn't easy, but it's not impossible either. Every human being experiences such losses, most of us many times over, so we have people all around us who can inspire us and offer gentle insight into how to make peace with change. By using Reiki and taking advantage of the spiritual wisdom of the principles, we can claim our own complete healing and be on our way to feeling happiness in our lives again, much sooner than we think.

REIKI FOR
A HEALTH PROBLEM

Several years ago, my friend Terry Graybill telephoned me with frightening news: her gynecologist had found a palpable mass in one of her breasts, and a mammogram had shown an amorphous calcium deposit in the other—warning signs of cancer. I drove to her house immediately so that I could comfort her and do Reiki.

We both recalled our teacher's encouragement to apply Reiki at the original site of infection or injury and to send Reiki to the original cause of a condition. If some situation had triggered negative feelings that had been repressed, resulting in "issues in the tissues," we were to support the client in identifying the situation and finding a healthy way to express those feelings. So Terry and I talked at length about what feelings she might have repressed that might now be showing up as medical problem.

Because breasts are associated with nurturing, and Terry has always "mothered" her cats, she considered the possibility that she had pent-up grief over the deaths of two of her elderly cats and three sick kittens she had adopted the previous year. To express the suppressed sadness, she decided that she would do quick crayon drawings each day, post them on her refrigerator, and then call me to talk about the drawings and how she felt. Meanwhile, she and her husband would do Reiki hands-on healing, and friends would send Reiki each day, to help prepare for further diagnostic tests. Having this treatment plan in place calmed Terry's immediate fears and helped her accept the reality that healing had already begun.

True to her word, she picked up the crayons each day and drew to express her sadness and fears: in one drawing, ghost cats floated above her as she lay prone on an operating table; in another, one of her cats rode a rocket to heaven. She found herself feeling the sadness she had suppressed for so long and letting it go. Soon she felt her sense of humor returning, and with it, her whole state of mind brightened like sunshine burning through the clouds. During the same period, she also received Reiki, which brought her healing on all levels.

When Terry drove to the hospital for the biopsy scheduled three weeks later, two girlfriends came with her for company and sent Reiki to her throughout the procedure. When she emerged from the outpatient testing area, though teary eyed from being stuck with needles, she had good news: the palpable mass had turned out to be merely a benign, fluid-filled sac.

She continued to do her crayon drawings and receive Reiki hands-on and distant healing. When the second diagnostic procedure was performed six weeks after the establishment of her Reiki treatment plan, the results were even more remarkable: radiologists had taken hundreds of digital images of her breast tissue, looking for the problematic calcium mass, but it had disappeared. They now found only a normal distribution.

When we use Reiki for a worrisome health problem, we can apply it in many ways: we can use both hands-on and distant healing; we can direct distant healing not only to the client but to the situation; and we can send Reiki forward in time to any scheduled tests, outpatient procedures, or surgeries. When we also use the common sense tools of creative expression, talking to a trusted friend, or therapy to process suppressed feelings that have begun to manifest as physical tension, discomfort, or disease, we create a new foundation for complete health and well-being.

Sometimes, even after a practitioner has considered an illness as an expression of suppressed feelings and then acknowledged and expressed those feelings, there's one more step: to identify the situation that triggered the illness and resolve it in a way that promotes well-being. This resolution may require that we forgive others who are or have been important in our lives; sometimes it requires that we forgive ourselves; and often it requires both. The work of Louise Hay (mentioned earlier in this book), who healed herself of cancer by exploring the relationship between her mind and body, learning to forgive, and becoming a positive thinker, can be thought provoking and helpful to anyone interested in exploring these ideas about the nature of illness, health, and well-being. Her story was made into a feature-length film, *You Can Heal Your Life*, after the book of the same name.

In addition to this work on emotional healing, the practitioner may want to learn some new communication or problem-solving skills to cope with the situation that initially triggered the illness. A psychotherapist or life coach may be able to offer excellent suggestions for improving communication skills. A close circle of friends may be willing and eager to brainstorm to discover solutions to more practical problems. Both of these strategies—processing feelings and problem solving—work for anyone, Reiki practitioner or not, and represent a healthy response to change, challenge, crisis, and the ongoing stresses of daily life. They help people cultivate more conscious awareness of their experiences, and empower people to adapt well to change, both through their own individual efforts and through the support of their communities.

NOW YOU:
APPLY REIKI AND PROCESS OR PROBLEM-SOLVE

As a Reiki practitioner, you're probably already well aware of the many ways that Reiki helps you to feel physically better each day. You know that Reiki relaxes tension, relieves pain, and accelerates healing, and you may have experienced Reiki's benefits in other ways as well.

When you're faced with a health problem of your own, use Reiki and consider using some form of creative expression to process the thoughts and feelings that you've repressed as unacceptable. By writing in a journal, drawing, painting, sculpting, making music, or dancing, you can safely explore your thoughts and feelings about your body and its health. What will emerge first on paper or in your composition are the thoughts and feelings you already hold in conscious awareness. Once these are expressed, others will surface from the subconscious that may seem new and surprising—or even shocking. Allow these thoughts and feelings to surface, however much you might want to censor them, and then gently, gradually explore their origins. These may be the very thoughts and feelings that now hold you back by creating discomfort or disease in your physical body so that you'll pay them some attention.

As you let these feelings emerge, and acknowledge and express them, notice your body. See how your shoulders relax and your posture becomes more erect. Feel how your breathing changes. Sense how your heart opens up, perhaps just a little, as you allow yourself to enjoy the conscious awareness that you're free of that sadness or worry, that disappointment or dread.

Sometimes, when we engage in journaling or other creative expression, memories begin to emerge that may feel too painful to explore. If this happens to you, *stop.* Consider contacting a therapist or counselor to ask for help in going further with your exploration. If you decide you would rather not seek professional support, at least make sure that a friend or loved one is available to listen and to support you as you express rage, grief, or sorrow. When we release such long-suppressed feelings, there is certainly relief, but often, there is also a renewed awareness of vulnerability. Another person can offer caring presence, which brings comfort. If this person can offer Reiki, so much the better! If not, do Reiki self-treatment, both hands-on and in the energy field, to help yourself to heal and claim closure.

As you might guess, the best way to avoid repressing emotions into the body is to acknowledge and express them as they arise. Committing to an ongoing journal or another form of creative expression is an excellent way to vent "unacceptable" feelings. When you sketch a little each day, you'll discover that an occasional, deliberately ugly drawing is a great way to dump unhappy feelings that have been knocking around inside. Plus, over time you'll hone an ability or talent for writing, art, music, or dance into a skill that gives you pleasure and brings you some peace of mind. That's a pretty good return on a small, daily investment of time!

REIKI FOR
WORRIES ABOUT
LARGE-SCALE DISASTERS

To the individual mind, even just one of the environmental issues we face seems enough to confound our problem-solving ability. What can we do, we wonder, to reverse global warming, the melting of the ice caps, and all the havoc with the world's weather that this ecological imbalance creates? And we recognize, of course, that the earth needs healing not only on the physical level but on the mental, emotional, and spiritual levels as well. How can we help to heal the ongoing war in Iraq or ease the suffering of those in Darfur who have survived "ethnic cleansing"? Such thoughts may tempt us beyond worry to depression and despair.

In the face of the world's many woes, saying "Just for today, do not worry" may seem more like denial than it does spiritual practice. However, when we accompany remembrance of the principles with Reiki healing, the possibility of saving the earth becomes real. The inscription on the Usui Memorial outside Saihoji Temple in Tokyo concludes with this remarkable expression of hope: "If Reiki can be spread throughout the world it will touch the human heart and the morals of society. It will be helpful for many people, and will not only heal disease, but also the earth as a whole."[4]

Now, just over eighty years later, we stand at that moment of opportunity: Reiki has spread worldwide. For decades, Reiki has been slowly, gently healing us. Many Reiki practitioners have witnessed miracles. Can we take the next step? Through our commitment to Reiki practice and to daily reflection on the Reiki principles, can we affect human morality? Can we bring about healing of "the earth as a whole"?

Experience with Reiki teaches us that the Reiki energy taps an infinite—and infinitely powerful—source of healing, the same source that Hawayo Takata sometimes called "God-power." Knowing that we are attuned to Reiki, and that it flows through and radiates outward from us, we may feel encouraged to believe that healing of "the earth as a whole" is possible. Grateful for this chance to offer healing, and releasing the outcome for the highest good, we figuratively roll up our sleeves, preparing to begin. But where do we start? What can we do?

Besides committing to practice Reiki on ourselves and offer it to others among our family and friends who are open to it, we can send Reiki distant healing to "the earth as a whole" and specific regions of the globe that are in upheaval.* A simple way to send Reiki healing, without using any symbols at all, is to raise your Reiki-charged hands to heart level, spread them a few inches apart with the palms facing each other, and imagine the earth between them. Say a prayer for the earth's healing and then just listen to your hands, lowering them when the flow of energy finally stops. Or, if

---

*Practitioners who wish to participate in a more organized effort to send Reiki healing to the earth may want to volunteer for Reiki Outreach International (www.annieo.com/reikioutreach). Another option is to use the World Peace Crystal Grids, placed by Reiki Master William Rand at the poles and in Jerusalem, as focal points for distant healing. Photos of the grids are posted online at www.reiki.org/GlobalHealing/Northandsouthpolehomepage.html.

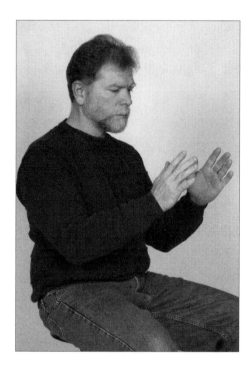

Rather than worry about the state of the world, send Reiki for earth healing.

you're not comfortable with saying a prayer, simply open your heart and send your love along with the Reiki energy. Listen to the flow, and lower your hands when it ceases.

Being able to take constructive action to resolve any problem, even one as multifaceted as the global environmental crisis or war in the Middle East, relieves some of the anxiety the problem evokes. Knowing that millions of other people are also engaged in the daily work of praying for peace and sending Reiki for earth healing also lightens the burden. When we all do our part in this way, remembering "Just for today, do not worry" seems to be a way to encourage ourselves and others to go on, though the road before us may be long and healing "the earth as a whole" may take generations.

SERENITY

Sometimes reciting the Reiki principle, "Just for today, do not worry," may not seem like enough to shift us from high anxiety to mental calm. However, when we combine it with committed Reiki practice, we can dissolve anxiety and claim not only calm but also peace of mind and trust in the healing power of

Source, which flows through our very capable hands. This is enough to help us confront our concerns and cope with them with intelligence and wisdom, making it possible to live each day with greater contentment and confidence, and to meet each day's challenges with serenity.

SUMMARY

When attuned to Reiki, we are empowered to bring healing through our hands to ourselves and others, healing that's not simply physical but also mental, emotional, and spiritual in nature. At the same time, we are seeded with an enlightened awareness cultivated simply through the practice of hands-on and distant healing, which teaches us compassion and the unwavering presence of a higher power whose nature is intelligent, loving, and kind. When practitioners combine committed Reiki practice with daily remembrance of the Reiki principles, they discover that they're blessed with some extraordinary resources for facing the challenges of everyday life.

As practitioners heal on all levels, they find that they make better choices when facing change. More often, they choose to express their feelings rather than repress them. They become more comfortable facing problems than avoiding them or denying their existence. They think about how they respond to challenging situations and recognize when they're using past behavior patterns rather than being fully present in the moment.

Like those who aren't trained in Reiki, practitioners often find psychotherapy, hypnosis, and metaphysical studies helpful in healing unhealthy behavior patterns they learned in response to past stresses or crises. Psychotherapy works by providing a venue for long-term, conscious exploration of feelings evoked by present-day challenges and past memories. Hypnosis and hypnotherapy directly reprogram the subconscious mind to healthier behavior through repeated suggestions; sometimes, deliberate reframing of traumatic past events in more positive terms is also used to facilitate forgiveness of the past and to safely release painful feelings. Metaphysics, positive thinking, and affirmative prayer offer many tools, including visualizations, treasure maps, and repeated affirmations, to shift consciousness and bring about positive changes of all kinds.

The effectiveness of such techniques for healing and spiritual development is enhanced by the use of Reiki. However, the practice of Reiki itself changes consciousness, because it brings healing on all levels to the practitioner as well as to the client. Eventually, with or without conscious effort to change unhealthy behavior patterns in response to stress, at least some of these patterns simply fall away, dissolved by years of exposure to Reiki Light.

What remains to be healed? This is an excellent question for Reiki practitioners to ask themselves as they continue to do hands-on and distant healing year after year, decade after decade. In the early years of practice, it may seem beside the point as we focus on healing physical complaints and restoring the body to its natural state of harmony and balance. Later on, however, when we're enjoying greater health and well-being, it makes sense to ask these questions: What remains to be healed within me on the emotional, mental, or spiritual level? What tasks do I avoid? Whose company do I dislike? What makes me feel worried? What unhealthy behavior patterns remain in my consciousness that Reiki might heal with a bit of effort on my part?

If we're willing to allow ourselves to consider these questions and answer them honestly, we'll come to a more conscious understanding of ourselves. Knowing how much Reiki has already healed us, we may work to heal any remaining emotional, mental, and spiritual wounds with confidence that we will ultimately succeed—and in doing so, come nearer to our own happiness.

Remembering the second Reiki principle, "Just for today, do not worry," may help us face our own need for deeper healing with humility, compassion, and trust in the power of Reiki itself. We may be recalled to calm serenity by reciting this principle morning and night. We may repeat it to ourselves in crisis and discover that it helps us remember to breathe, relax our bodies, and move forward with balance and grace. We may even find that our intention to live by this principle shifts us into a higher state of consciousness so that we meet the day with mindfulness, observing the challenges before us with sufficient detachment from them to make sound choices, guided by both common sense and that unconditionally loving higher intelligence that we experience when we do Reiki and connect to the Source of all healing and life itself.

MORE SUGGESTIONS FOR PRACTICE

❧ When you practice Reiki on yourself or a client, let your mind become naturally quiet. Notice the energy flowing through your hands. Trace the energy back to Source as far as you can. Appreciate the healing flow. Let the act of doing Reiki become your entrance into spiritual sanctuary.

❧ Remember the Reiki principles each day, recalling them in the morning before you set off for work and at night before you go to bed. Let them anchor you in the intention to be spiritually guided. When you feel faced with a crisis, silently repeat "Just for today, do not worry" to yourself like a mantra. Don't let anyone or anything move you out of your own calm center without your conscious consent.

❧ Feeling overwhelmed? Surrender the load you're carrying on your shoulders. Use prayer and meditation to turn over your concerns to Spirit. Use Reiki to calm yourself down and clear your mind. Be open to the possibility of inner guidance coming to you in a word, an image, a knowing without knowing how you know. Be grateful when you receive such guidance and honor it. If you begin to feel uncertain, confused, or anxious again, go back into meditation and prayer. Learn to live a Spirit-guided life.

❧ Learn healthy coping mechanisms rather than relying on knee-jerk, unhealthy behaviors learned in the past. Can you mentally reframe the issues that concern you so that they're reduced from movie-screen size to wallet-photo size? This is an actual technique used by practitioners of Neuro-Linguistic Programming to help their clients to see problems as manageable rather than overwhelming. Can you schedule ten minutes of worry time at 5:15 p.m. rather than let worry run through you like a slow poison all day long at work? Can you imagine the worst-case scenario for a situation that concerns you, accept it, and recognize that even if such an unlikely outcome were to occur, you have the inner resources to cope? Can you make the complex project seem more doable by mentally breaking it down into much smaller parts? Can you take physical breaks, like a trip to the gym at lunchtime, to relieve the tension in your body? Can you take mental breaks, like ten minutes of daydreaming about your next vacation, to refresh your mind? Can you take a Reiki break, wherever you are, to relax your physical body and dissolve any feelings of anxiety? All of these strategies can help reduce your stress.

❧ To stay on an even keel emotionally, engage in some creative activity on a daily basis, even if just for a short time. Let your purpose be to engage with the form and express what you feel rather than to produce something perfect (because that goal can become a source of stress). Just write out your anxiety. Just dance out your fury. Be with your feelings, good, bad, and ugly—and let them out into the light of day, where you can see and reflect on them, and, if necessary, let them go. You'll find that you feel better—and your mind is so much clearer!

❧ Scale the mountain, as Mikao Usui did. Recognize whatever it is that you need to do and then do it, putting all worry aside as you begin. Do what is right, and knowing that it's right, don't let anxiety or doubt enter your mind. Treat such feelings as unwelcome houseguests. If you see worry coming, lock the door, close the curtains, and go out the back way—but *do* go on.

❧ Let your moments of success give you lasting confidence. After a friend invited me to go "bouldering" with him in a state park and I found that I had climbed a 120-foot-high cliff, I experienced an amazing aftereffect: for the next year and a half, I was convinced that I could do almost anything. To climb the cliff, I had to surrender my fear of heights at the base, trust my friend to rig the climbing gear correctly, and trust Spirit. I did it! I was so surprised at my sense of accomplishment. What successes have you had that required you to put aside a fear? Make a list. When you are faced with something that challenges you, look at that list again. Can you see how the person who accomplished the items on that list has the inner resources to face the situation before you now? Yes, you can.

❧ Be inspired by the stories of others who have faced difficult life challenges to face your own challenges. Think about the lives of Mikao Usui, Chujiro Hayashi, and Hawayo Takata. Their lives were not always easy or worry free. Yet they lived by the Reiki principles and recognized the power of the energy to bring healing into every aspect of their lives. The lives of other Reiki practitioners may inspire you as well, although courage and inner strength can be found all around us, in people everywhere. Choose to imitate people who demonstrate peace, serenity, gratitude, integrity, and kindness.

Recognize your own inner strength and courage, but don't be afraid to ask for support and help from people who care about you. Reiki friends are often inspired and guided when they make helpful suggestions. Asking another Reiki practitioner or a community of practitioners to send Reiki to you or to your situation multiplies the healing effort and the healing effects many times over. Be grateful for such support, and don't hesitate to ask for it. The energy does the healing, but most Reiki practitioners are very glad to be able to help.

5

GRATITUDE

"Be Grateful: Show Appreciation"

The third Reiki principle encourages us to feel gratitude for our lives, from first breath to last, and every breath between. In the most recent translations from the Japanese, we are advised: "Be grateful. Show appreciation." However, Takata's comments on this principle encourage us to apply it to every aspect of our lives. We are to find ways to show our respect, affection, and appreciation for everything and everyone that nurtures and supports us, from the earth and the elements of nature to our elders and ancestors.

When we're thankful for a new day, for the first notes of bird song, for the dawn, for the sight of our sleepy faces looking back at us in the mirror, we're acknowledging the quality of our own lives and appreciating whatever force in the universe brings such moments into our lives. What we call this force doesn't matter; many names have been used: Creator, Spirit, Source, Jehovah, God, Allah, and even Universal Life-Force Energy. Whatever we call this force, when we acknowledge our dependence on it—for life, shelter, sustenance, family and friends, all blessings—and simply feel thankful, our gratitude restores

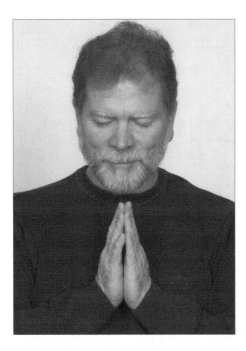

Practicing gratitude

us to a childlike spiritual innocence. This restoration of spiritual innocence makes it possible for us to be in the world with a new, or renewed, sense of purpose and to move forward in hope and faith.

Experiencing gratitude, we can feel at home in the world yet not of it; we can feel that our lives are as secure, and insecure, as anyone's, and yet have the confidence that our lives are in the hands of God; we can be content with our lives just as they are, knowing that the past is healing and the future is full of wonderful opportunities. For the experience of gratitude is on the way—and all along the way—to peace. Only when we begin to welcome gratitude into our lives with every breath do we discover that it opens the door to well-being and happiness.

How can we practice gratitude? Most people begin by counting their blessings. For a Reiki practitioner, Reiki itself may be the first blessing that comes to mind. Our journey may encompass not only celebration of the extraordinary healing that Reiki brings, which lights our way, but also grateful acknowledgment of the ordinary, which is then elevated to the sacred. Through conscious effort and daily practice, we can come to appreciate what we previously took for granted; what we thought was a burden, disappointment, or difficulty; what we considered a cross to bear—and have come to realize is a blessing in disguise.

This appreciation can transform our lives, inviting day-to-day contentment so that we feel touched by simple pleasure and joy.

REIKI TEACHES GRATITUDE

Gratitude is a feeling of awareness and appreciation for the good in our lives. For most of us, it's easy to be thankful for a special privilege or spiritual blessing, as Hawayo Takata was during her course of instruction by Dr. Hayashi on her way to teach Usui Reiki (as described in her diary entry of May 1936).

> What was more than pleasing was that Mr. Hayashi has granted to bestow upon me the secret of Shinpiden—Kokiyo-ho and the Leiji-ho—the utmost secret in the Energy Science. Know [sic] one can imagine my happiness to think that I have the honor and respect to be trusted with this gift—a gift of a lifetime . . .[1]

However, gratitude is good in itself, and the more gratitude we feel, the more conscious we are of being in "a state of grace."

Like Hawayo Takata, most of us feel very grateful when we learn Reiki, when we can continue our training, when we find we've built a regular client practice, when we receive support from a fellow practitioner in the form of a kind word or comforting touch, and most of all, when we are privileged to witness miracles. And since Reiki is "the miracle medicine for all diseases," according to the second of the two original titles for the Reiki principles, miracles happen for all of us sooner or later.

In June 2007, Aimee Kovac, a newly initiated practitioner, wrote:

> Thank you so much. . . . I am *amazed* by what I've experienced doing Reiki just this past month. Not only has it been beneficial for my husband's diabetes, but . . . I've worked on my son as well; the Reiki has alleviated his headache and settled his stomach. It greatly reduced pain he was having in his ankle after twisting it. At this point, they're both asking for treatments whenever there's a need. . . . It is a blessing to witness the subtle workings of the universe on a regular basis![2]

Gratitude lays the foundation of the path many practitioners walk with Reiki: gratitude for Reiki, for a friend or relative who is open minded enough to try it, for the opportunity to offer it to a client, for the healing that occurs, and for the lessons learned about the nature of healing. Gratitude does this for many practitioners, even though at first we might feel it only as a fleeting awareness: "This is a good experience; I'm glad to be here and able to offer Reiki."

The more we practice Reiki hands-on and distant healing, the more we experience what amazes and delights us, the more we notice our own improving sense of well-being, and the more we realize that we can have a positive and meaningful impact on the world. Our gratitude deepens. We begin to wonder more often about the source of Reiki energy healing. What does it mean to channel universal or Spirit-guided life-force energy? Gradually, we come to understand that the energy is both healer and teacher, and the lesson we are learning is one of unconditional love. Our hearts open even more, and we move through gratitude to joy.

EARLY PRACTICE OF GRATITUDE

Most Reiki practitioners taught in the Western tradition (Usui Shiki Ryoho) learn of the Reiki principles during their level I class, either through a series of brief meditations that precede the four attunements (acceptance, gratitude, integrity, and kindness) or through the presentation of Reiki history, which often occurs near the end of the class. Often, the Reiki principles are deliberately de-emphasized. A conscientious Reiki master might say, "Understand that these are not commandments or rules for right living. Reiki is simple, without doctrine or dogma. You are not required to memorize them or make them part of your everyday life. Mikao Usui chose to recite the principles as part of his daily meditation. Perhaps, at some point in your practice, you may want to do that as well. Just remembering the principles from time to time will help you make healthier choices—acceptance over anxiety or anger; gratitude instead of resentment, impatience, or envy; integrity over mediocrity; and kindness over indifference."

Because the Reiki principles are downplayed, most students begin their practice with a focus on doing Reiki and experiencing the healing energy flowing through their hands—and this is just as it should be. The time just after learning Reiki is like a long honeymoon with Spirit. Practitioners learn to use their hands with gratitude and grace, and are privileged to witness miracles.

Yet eventually, "real life"—ordinary, unconsecrated experience—intrudes. The boss keeps us so late at work to finish an important project that when we finally get home, we fall asleep on the couch in our clothes, forgetting to do Reiki. The next morning, we're so tired that we sleep through the alarm, so there's no time to do Reiki. Over the next few days, somehow the same thing happens again and again. When Friday arrives, we're grumpy and out of sorts—and the last thing we want to do is Reiki. Instead, we opt for happy hour or cut out of town for the beach. It's only after we've escaped to our old haunts and discovered that we don't feel quite as satisfied as we used to that we realize we haven't done Reiki in days. What will happen? Will we lose it?

We remember what it feels like to do Reiki: the quiet contentment of practice; the pleasure of our own bodies, humming with life; the joy in our ability to actually do something to help bring healing to another human being. And yes, we may remember—what were they called?—the Reiki principles. How do they begin? Oh, yes, "Just for today . . ." There's something forgiving of the past in that phrase, something that invites a renewed commitment in the present. We find a quiet corner, lean back, place our hands in first position, close our eyes, and feel the flow. We savor and celebrate it, because we feel so grateful.

When we return home, we shuffle through papers and books until we find our class notes, and there they are—the Reiki principles: "Just for today, do not anger . . . do not worry . . . be grateful . . ." Be grateful? Well, we realize, sometimes that's going to be a challenge: after a hard work week, after a difficult conversation with a roommate, when we step in a puddle and ruin a pair of shoes, when we're stuck in an airport that's closed down because of the weather and our entire vacation is delayed. How can we begin to be grateful for experiences like *those?*

This becomes the question of the day and of the days that follow. As we find ourselves doing Reiki again each day, wondering why we ever stopped when it feels so good and does so much good, we think about gratitude. We go deeper in our practice and attempt to "count our blessings"—and the honeymoon with Spirit recommences. We integrate some of Reiki energy's subtle healing. We do memorize the Reiki principles, and when confronted with difficulties, we draw them forth like swords to slay our personal demons.

We may do this—practice Reiki, become distracted, feel our longing, and return—again and again until we know that what we want is more than just a honeymoon; we want the unconditional love that flows from Spirit into our hearts and through our hands when we do Reiki to be with us at every moment of every day of our lives. We want to do Reiki, and we want to remember the Reiki principles. We want this love to last a lifetime.

Do we feel grateful in the face of the prolonged suffering of someone we love? Do we feel a sense of appreciation when disaster strikes us? Can we recognize that death can be a blessing when we experience loss? No, we certainly can't—not at first, but after practicing the principle of gratitude, we begin to discover our own inner resources and to acknowledge and celebrate the support that we're offered from every direction. When we emerge from crisis, we discover that we've developed new strengths, found new friends, relied on Spirit—and fallen more deeply in love with life itself.

GRATITUDE IN
THE FACE OF DISASTER

Kay Sivel's clear blue eyes sparkle with warmth and kindness; her soft, silver hair flips up on her shoulders, framing a beautiful face; her tiny figure makes her seem almost fairylike, belying her inner strength. Fifteen years in substance abuse recovery have made her honest and forthcoming about her own feelings. She is also able to listen to others with sympathy and hear what they have to say without judgment. Kay learned Reiki in 2000 and quickly realized that it felt right to her: she wanted to pursue learning to the master level and be able to teach this natural method of healing to others in recovery, especially for *self*-healing. For those who had a history of choosing alcohol or drugs to numb the pain, Reiki could bring calm. She also wanted to learn Reiki for her dogs. For almost as long as she has been in recovery, she has bred and trained dogs. Recently, she added dog massage to the services she offers.

On the evening of Thursday, September 15, 2005, Kay received a telephone call from her son while she was in a meeting. "Mom," Paul said simply, "the house is on fire. I've got the dogs out. I've called the fire department, and the fire engines are on their way. I think you should come home."

Kay got off the phone, grabbed her purse and car keys, and ran to her car. She prayed during the twenty-minute drive home. She, her husband Jim, and her son Paul had only recently moved into the beautiful two-story house in the woods. Now it was going up in smoke and flames. What else could she do besides pray? She could send Reiki—and ask others to send Reiki.

By the time she arrived, fire engines already blocked her narrow gravel driveway. The firefighters were just starting to get the flames under control. The front of the house was charcoal, glowing embers, and ash, although the back still seemed to be standing. She felt too stunned even to cry.

She made two phone calls: one to her mother and one to me to ask for Reiki to be sent immediately to the situation. Then she stood back and watched the firefighters going in and out of the dark smoke and flames with their axes and hoses. The fire crackled and sparked in an absurd parody of the fires she and Jim had enjoyed in the living room fireplace of their home on winter evenings. The water in the hoses gushed and roared.

She felt too numb to be anxious or angry but realized that she did feel grateful. Her house was burning down, but her husband, a piano tuner, was at her side. Her son was alive and well, and safely away from the fire. A kind neighbor was now watching her beloved dogs. What had she lost really? Her beautiful house . . .

But a house could be rebuilt, possibly even better than before. She and Jim did have homeowner's insurance that would surely pay for the cost of any necessary repairs. Nothing truly important to her—not her husband, her son, or her animals—had been lost or even hurt or injured in the fire. She would count her blessings. She began to feel how fortunate she was as she watched the firefighters douse the last of the flames.

Before her stood a blackened, charred shell. The front half of her house had burned down, but the back stood a little out of kilter, like an unfinished backdrop for a play. Were there any possessions she should try to save? The firefighters wouldn't even let her look through the still-smoking rubble. *No, there's a lot that I'm just going to have to let go. 'Let go and let God,'* she thought.

The important thing is that everyone I love is safe, she told herself. *I am so grateful for that!* Holding this thought in her mind and heart for comfort, she walked to the neighbor's house to see her dogs—and to begin the work of finding somewhere to live.

For a few days Kay and Jim lived with relatives, who also supplied some clothes. (The master bedroom, which contained all their personal possessions, had been in the part of the house that burned down.) Eventually, their homeowner's insurance enabled them to rent a trailer, in which they lived for six months as their house was gradually rebuilt.

Kay loves her new house as much as the old one, perhaps even more. What she has taken away from the experience of the fire is a profound gratitude that her family was spared, a deeper awareness of her appreciation and love for each member of her family, and a renewed faith in humanity. She is thankful to all the neighbors, friends, and acquaintances who helped in whatever way they could. She is comforted by the knowledge that there were so many who stood by her through disaster, and has no doubt that they would again if she and her family faced other difficulties. "I have a lot to be grateful for," she says, with a bright smile.

NOW YOU:
PRACTICE EMOTIONAL ALCHEMY

Medieval alchemists strove to turn lead and other base metals into gold. When we face real disaster in our lives, it's quite natural to go into shock, feel numb, and then grieve: to deny our loss, rage at it, mourn it, and finally accept it.

Of course, Reiki can help us cope with personal disaster. It can soothe hurts, calm inner turmoil, and help us to heal in the most gentle way possible. All that's necessary is to remember to use our own Reiki-charged hands on ourselves—at the heart, on the lower rib cage over the adrenal glands, and over the solar plexus; it's also sensible and wise to ask others to do Reiki on us and to send Reiki to us and to those we love.

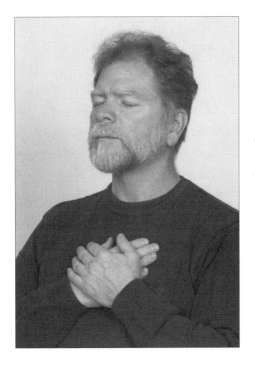

When faced with personal disaster or loss, do Reiki at the heart to bring calm—and practice gratitude.

We can also practice gratitude. Although the impact of any disaster is stunning, when we come to ourselves, we can look—and continue to look until we find—something good in the situation. This isn't easy. This is a spiritual accomplishment that requires conscious effort and the deliberate use of will to create change. However, this effort and intention enable us to transmute heavy, leaden feelings into bright, spiritual gold.

Gratitude sometimes requires an intentional adjustment of our vantage point to see the advantage point. To practice gratitude, look for—and find—the good that remains, despite what is gone. This deliberate practice of gratitude attracts more good. This is the work of spiritual alchemy: by choosing to look for and find something in a difficult situation for which we can feel grateful, we precipitate a series of changes: first, our own feelings begin to change from negative to positive; second, as we maintain our focus on gratitude, our sense of well-being improves, our personal energy levels increase, and our interactions with others begin to reflect this harmony; and finally, by continuing to focus our thoughts and feelings on the good in our lives, we draw more good into our lives. Sometimes this impacts the situation itself, making it possible for a more positive outcome to occur than we had imagined possible.

133

GRATITUDE FOR REIKI
AND THE HOPE OF HEALING

Shortly after Sharon Riegner completed her Reiki master training in June 2005, her mother-in-law died suddenly. Her husband Rick, who had loved his mother deeply, took the loss hard, and two weeks later he suffered a silent heart attack. His only symptom was mild indigestion after dinner one Friday night, something not remarkable in itself, even taking into account the stress of burying his mother and immediately returning to work. Sharon gave him hands-on Reiki, but after a couple of hours of treatment Rick still felt queasy so she called a few Reiki practitioner friends to ask them to send Reiki distant healing.

Rick's upset stomach seemed to subside as he relaxed at home that weekend, but when the alarm went off at 7 a.m. Monday morning, Sharon took one look at him, felt a wave of love and concern, and decided that she was going to insist that he see a doctor before going in to work. Although Rick said that he felt well enough to go to work, she argued that it was "better to be safe than sorry." She persuaded him to let her take him to a nearby hospital emergency room.

When Rick registered as a patient and described his single symptom of mild, persistent indigestion to the nurses on duty, they were not overly concerned. Perhaps he had experienced a gallbladder attack. However, one nurse anticipated the attending physician's probable orders. She prepped Rick for an electrocardiogram and ran the test herself. As soon as the picture began to emerge of the unsteady, rapid beating of his heart, she set off at a run, calling for a doctor to come *now*. Almost sixty hours after Rick's first complaint he was diagnosed: he was undergoing a silent heart attack.

At his side, Sharon continued to do Reiki. Even though she was stunned by this terrible news, she determined to think of it in the most positive terms. Rather than wondering why Reiki had not prevented Rick's heart attack, she chose to believe that Reiki had helped keep him alive through the weekend. She dared to hope that it had minimized the damage to his heart as well. As her heart filled with gratitude for the blessing of Reiki, she began to feel more at peace. With half her attention on the medical personnel rushing to prepare her husband for immediate surgery, she sent him more Reiki, and she prayed.

In the operating room, a surgeon inserted a catheter and four surgical stints to open one completely blocked artery. Following this emergency procedure, more diagnostic tests were performed. These revealed more severely clogged arteries and a tear in the lower part of the heart that was quickly developing into a heart aneurysm. Rick's heart was so damaged that his physicians recommended a heart transplant—a surgery that they were neither willing nor equipped to perform at their hospital. The prognosis was even more unsettling: the doctors felt that Rick was unlikely to survive.

Rick remained in the hospital for two weeks, until his vital signs stabilized enough that he could be transferred to a large city hospital fifty miles away. During this time, Sharon was constantly at his bedside doing Reiki. Sometimes other Reiki practitioners visited to join in the hands-on healing effort. Meanwhile, many people sent distant healing. Both Sharon and Rick are convinced that this focused healing effort had a powerful impact on his prognosis.

Once he was transferred, more diagnostic tests were performed. Rick's physician had good news for them: he did not need a heart transplant, his aneurysm could be repaired by a cardiac surgeon on staff, and his chances of survival and full recovery were very good, estimated to be about 94 percent. Relief brought tears to Sharon's eyes. She reached for her husband's hand and smiled at him with renewed hope.

Rick was immediately scheduled for open-heart surgery. Just a month after he had lost his mother, he lay on the operating table for the second time. During the operation cardiac surgeons inspected and determined more exactly the extent of the damage to his heart. They decided to leave the four surgical stints that had already been inserted in place. Then they repaired the aneurysm with a patch, did a double bypass on two partially blocked arteries to prevent future trouble, and closed up.

Hours later, after Rick had recovered consciousness and been wheeled back to his room in Cardiac ICU, his heart went into atrial fibrillation. Although Rick's nurses told Sharon that this was fairly common after open-heart surgery, she still had a very difficult time watching the heart monitors above his bed trace the wild and erratic rhythms of his heart over the next six hours. Nurses monitored his condition closely and administered medication, and Sharon and her friend and fellow Reiki Master Barbara Sautter gave Rick hands-on healing. A nurse reassured them with a few kind words: "He's doing fantastically well, considering what he's been through." Finally, his heart settled in a steady, healthy rhythm, and from that point on his recovery proceeded without any further incidents.

Two weeks after Rick was released from the hospital he and Sharon returned for a follow-up visit. When they asked his doctor for more information about the extent of the damage to Rick's heart from the heart attack, he told them, "It's minimal. Go live your lives. You can do whatever you want." This was news for rejoicing. They both felt deeply grateful for the miracle of healing that had occurred in their lives as a result of Rick's treatment with excellent allopathic medical care and countless hours of Reiki.

Rick followed his physician's recommendation to wait six months before returning to full-time work (a normal recovery period for open-heart surgery). During this time, Rick and Sharon talked often about the transformative power of healing and about ways to carry its positive effects forward into the rest of their lives. Often, they told one another how grateful they were for all the blessings they had already shared. Their love for one another deepened, and now their marriage seems stronger and happier. They have both changed their eating habits and lost weight. They now take yoga classes together. Rick became Sharon's first Reiki student, and this, too, has brought them closer.

Sharon says, "I am so grateful for Reiki. I know the heart does respond to love—and that's what Reiki is: unconditional love. It has brought both our hearts tremendous healing." In the moment of greatest crisis, she made the choice to see Reiki as keeping Rick alive and moderating the damage during a silent heart attack. She allowed herself to feel grateful for this healing. This choice—and her practice of gratitude—opened the way for greater healing and, ultimately, for Rick's complete recovery.

NOW YOU:
SEE THE GLASS AS HALF-FULL

Although it takes time—and experience—to learn to trust that Reiki does indeed bring healing to the whole person and that the energy works in harmony with nature and allopathic medicine for the highest good, when you do Reiki, be grateful for whatever healing occurs. Instead of wishing that the Reiki you've done were more effective or more fast-acting, be glad for whatever reduction in pain or other symptoms you observe.

During a Reiki treatment, pay attention to whatever thoughts cross your mind; in the aftermath of a treatment, notice your passing thoughts as well. If it occurs to you that you might need to go to the doctor for a checkup or that you should advise your client to see a doctor, do so. Reiki can help us to heal in many ways, not only by providing immediate pain and symptom relief. Sometimes it works by moderating symptoms, prompting an awareness of the need for medical treatment, and supporting accelerated healing during medical treatment. Be grateful that Reiki can bring hidden chronic conditions to light for healing.

GRATITUDE PLUS DETERMINATION EQUALS SUCCESS

When Karen Thompson walks into a room, people turn their heads as if suddenly aware of a ray of sunshine. The pretty redhead with the bright smile is a psychotherapist who works primarily with children from homes where there's drug or alcohol addiction. Karen is also a survivor of radiation and thyroid removal for Graves' disease. She has been told that she will be on thyroid medication for the rest of her life.

Learning Reiki inspired her to take better care of herself. In addition to making time for an occasional massage or other bodywork, she decided to become a triathlete. She knew that the exercise would help her relax workday tensions and lose weight; she also wanted the sense of accomplishment that would come from fulfilling a cherished dream.

In November 2005, shortly after beginning her Reiki master training, she began training for a triathlon set for July 2006. On a regular basis, she made time to run and bike along the Perkiomen Creek Park trails, and swim laps at the local Y. As she continued to train month after month, she found that she felt more vital and healthy than she had in years. She lost close to ten pounds and liked the way her clothes fit. She admired the athletic look of her body.

She felt pleased with herself, proud of her ability to make and keep a commitment to her own health, and grateful for the support of Reiki friends who had sent distant healing to help her achieve her goal. She felt psychologically and physically ready to compete.

About two weeks before the triathlon, a freak summer storm drummed down rain, flooding the creek and submerging long stretches of the roads near her home. Venturing out after the downpour, she tried to drive her SUV through rushing water that was several inches deep. Instead, her SUV was swept off the road and into a drainage ditch in the strong current. She was hurled forward by the impact so that her face was bruised against the windshield and her ribs abraded by the seat belt. After getting out of the vehicle into water covering rough terrain, she fell, cutting and bruising her legs as well.

Two days later, she attended a Reiki healing circle that began with a verbal check-in. Karen introduced herself and then struggled not to cry as she explained how her face came to be swollen, one eye shadowed by a bruise, and her legs covered with healing cuts. "I don't think I'll be able to run this race," she said in a little girl voice. "It's only eight days away."

"We'll send Reiki," several people said at once.

She swallowed hard, searching the eyes of everyone in the healing circle, and nodded. "Thanks," she said simply, and then again, "Thanks."

She took her turn on a bodywork table that afternoon and received a thorough Reiki treatment from those present. Promised the support of daily distant healing by so many people, she pushed herself to begin training again, going a fraction of her usual distance but increasing it each day. On July 30, 2006, she competed in her first triathlon meet, beat her own "personal best" time—and her brother, much to his surprise. Her sense of victory was colored by gratitude to everyone who had supported her with Reiki, kind words, and gentle encouragement.

NOW YOU:
USE GRATITUDE TO
FACE DOWN YOUR DEMONS

One of the most difficult spiritual challenges is when circumstances outside your control divert you from your chosen course or the goal you want to accomplish. It's easy to feel defeated by life itself when such obstacles are put in your way. It is tempting to indulge in hours of self-pity, which can deepen into days of depression. It's also tempting to rail against life's unfairness to anyone who will listen. This, too, can become something darker: enduring bitterness and resentment, which are slow-acting spiritual poisons.

When you're faced with a difficulty that you couldn't have anticipated, remember that just for today, just for this moment, you have a choice: to be grateful for every step forward you've been able to make toward your goal, even if now you must set it aside. You can be glad for every single ounce of strength you've gained, even if you think you'll never be able to train again. You can appreciate all the progress you've been able to make in developing your talent and abilities, despite the detour in your career path that life now sets before you. If you choose to be grateful for all that you've been able to accomplish so far and for all the support you've received, you will find a new respect for your own inner resources, you'll discover that you can handle the deferment of your own desires, and you may be happily surprised: what you have given up as impossible may again become possible, if not immediately, then another day.

ON THE WAY TO GRATITUDE

I was seated on the aisle of a "puddle jumper," one of those tiny commuter jets designed to cost-effectively transport business executives to meetings in other cities and states. The plane held perhaps a dozen people altogether, including the pilots and flight attendants. There was no legroom and scarcely any elbow room. As we prepared for takeoff, the February sky visible outside the little rectangle of window was a cold and threatening gray, and I was trying to control my fear of flying into snow or a storm.

This was a relatively recent phobia. For most of my adult life, I had enjoyed flying. I was happy to take in the view during the plane's ascension and then retreat into a book or magazine. However, since a death in the family in January 2004, I've felt less anchored to the earth, less sure of my safety here. In dreams since then, I've driven up a bridge ramp and awakened with my heart pounding as the car teetered at the edge of empty space; I've been a nervous traveler in a "Chunnel" train, all too aware of the pressure of water above; I've been the panicked plane passenger who pounded on the exit door to be let out, despite the fact that the plane flew thirty thousand feet in the air. Now, on this necessary flight, awake and alert, I forced myself to let go of my tense grip on the seat arms and rest my hands in my lap. Discreetly, I hoped to saturate myself with Reiki.

But I had to unbuckle my seat belt and get up to admit the passenger booked for the window seat beside me. He was a large man, who excused himself as he clambered past me, then quickly stashed his carry-on bag and sat down. As soon as he buckled up, he thrust a hand at me and introduced himself with a pronounced Southern drawl. "I'm Jackson Davis," he said. "My mama named me after two heroes of the War Between the States, but don't mind that. That's my name, but that's not my war."

He looked as if he could have been a Civil War soldier, despite what he said. He wore his red hair shorn close to his head, but his sideburns were long and blended into a neatly trimmed beard. He was fair skinned and freckled, with light blue-gray eyes that would have looked good with a Confederate soldier's uniform.

I introduced myself to him and asked if he'd ever flown that route before. (I was trying not to confess my fear of flying.)

"All the time," he said, shifting in his seat so that he blocked more of the view out the window. "I'm a computer consultant for a trucking company headquartered near here, so I'm back and forth between here and Savannah a couple times a month." Behind him, the view out the window angled upward slightly. I realized that we'd taken off, and I relaxed just a little bit. I already felt grateful that I was seated beside a friendly stranger. I thought of all the Reiki energy I had sent forward in time to calm myself down enough to take the flight and all the energy I had asked others to send. I felt the warmth of my hands through the seatbelt. Maybe I *could* do this.

For the next three hours, Jackson and I continued talking. I learned a lot about computerization in eighteen- and twenty-four-wheel trucks. I heard about his business and his family. I listened to him describe his house on a lake in northern Georgia and his favorite toy, a cigarette boat that he loved to speed across the water. He learned a little about me too—enough to reassure me of the statistical safety of flying. By the time we landed, I was convinced that

Spirit had sent me an angel disguised as a man to keep me company through the flight. His "assignment" was simply to distract me from my worries. He succeeded, and instead of feeling anxious, I felt gratitude for the duration of the flight. I thanked him for his good company and conversation, and we parted. I was quite sure that I would never see him again.

I made my way through the airport to the next gate, where a huge Boeing 747 would transport me to my final destination. I wasn't afraid anymore! I still felt touched by this stranger's kindness, and comforted and uplifted by a sense of the energy's protection. I thought about the power of gratitude: like a strong, broad-shouldered man, it could push away worries and fears. It could open the door of a closed mind to a different worldview that encompassed new and wonderful possibilities.

Gratitude is a bit like New York's Grand Central Station. You can get there from almost anywhere and arrive in any condition, but once there, you can change trains. If you've arrived on a mental and emotional "train" of anger and frustration, you can get off and go into gratitude, spend a little time there, and in a half hour or so, catch a different "train" for that desirable country location, peace of mind. If you've arrived on a "train" of anxiety, worry, and fear, you can go into gratitude, find some refreshment, and, when you are ready, leave on foot, feeling calm and optimistic once more.

Gratitude has the capacity to transform our experience in a positive way in a very short time. We may gravitate toward it naturally in crisis, or we may not, but even if not, we can still *choose* to enter gratitude. It can be a way station that we pass through on our way to another feeling, or it can be a destination in itself.

A STEP TOWARD GRATITUDE

It was just one of those days. Although I began the day with my usually comforting routine of a cup of coffee, writing in a journal, and doing Reiki, I found that I couldn't get down to work. I sat at my desk but couldn't focus. By midday, I felt frustrated with my lack of progress and worried that I was wasting time. I decided to take a walk to clear my head. I checked the thermostat outside the back door. On this particular January afternoon, the temperature hovered around thirty-five degrees Fahrenheit, and there was a cold, raw wind. I went back inside to put on a long, hooded coat; hid the lower half of my face behind a ski mask; wrapped a scarf around my neck; and pulled on earmuffs, a hat, and insulated gloves. Although I knew I might look strange to passersby, I was ready, and I would be warm. I pulled the front door firmly closed behind me, slipped my house keys into a pocket, and set off at a brisk pace.

Quickly, I found my stride, my arms swinging in thick arcs as I walked the gray road. I could see my breath. Then I couldn't see anything at all, because the cloud of air I had exhaled rose up from under the ski mask to fog my glasses. I stopped, cleaned off the lenses with a tissue, put my glasses back on, and began to walk again. This went on for about ten minutes, until I warmed up enough to pull off the ski mask. Once that happened, I could see where I was going—not a necessity, since my feet knew the way, but a simple pleasure. On this wintry day, the sky was mother-of-pearl gray, with a slur of clouds that mostly hid the sun, which seemed spectral, cold, and far away. The fields were dull and the trees bare, with the exception of some tall, majestic evergreens in the far distance. There was a penetrating silence.

I walked on, determined to cover the usual distance, despite the cold and gloom of the day. My turning point is usually a one-lane bridge over the west branch of the Perkiomen Creek. On this winter day, looking out at the black water of the creek, still edged with tiny shoals of ice and snow, didn't appeal to me. Instead, I turned off the road before the bridge to climb the hill into the woods. I trudged upward, my boots heavy, paused to catch my breath at intervals, and stopped long enough to read the yellow NO TRESPASSING signs posted on one of the trees. Only once before had I encroached on this land, and on that day, I had seen deer darting into the woods three times along the way.

At the crest of the hill, I dodged barbed wire and brush to get onto a wide trail that runs parallel to a narrow border of evergreen trees that seem destined for future Christmases. In my heavy coat and boots, I felt clumsy. I knew that I couldn't walk quietly, however much I tried. As I had expected, I saw no wildlife, not even a squirrel or a rabbit. I felt my disappointment as an added weight.

Then my mind returned to the Reiki principles, particularly to gratitude.

Once before, within the past few weeks, I had recognized the burden of negative emotion that I was carrying like a load on my back, unable to set it down. I had decided to write in my journal, not to vent but to express gratitude. The few minutes that I spent writing, "I am grateful for my life. I am grateful for the blessing of Reiki. I am grateful for . . . ," had shifted my mood and energy. Instead of feeling bogged down, overwhelmed, and incompetent, gratitude had helped me recognize that I am buoyed up by the universe, blessed with wonderful opportunities, and capable of taking advantage of them.

Remembering how effective this simple journal exercise had been, I decided that I would try it again when I got back to the house. Then it occurred to me that I didn't have to wait until I had finished my walk to change my mind and mood. I could start thinking thoughts of gratitude *now*. The day did not change; it stayed cold, dull gray, and gloomy. Instead, something in me changed—my attitude, my intention, and my willingness to do the spiritual work. Suddenly, I was aware that inside my coat pockets, my gloved hands radiated Reiki energy that penetrated through all the layers of clothing to warm my ribs and the cold breath in my lungs.

I laughed out loud. What a revelation! The practice of the Reiki principles invites the energy. It seemed almost like a mathematical formula in its precision: put one practitioner in a difficult situation or frame of mind, then add the practitioner's commitment to focus on gratitude, and the end result is a sudden release of healing energy, available to be put to good use.

Slowly, I descended the hill, still following the rough trail that paralleled the fir trees. A lone birdcall sounded, breaking the silence. A single stand of dried summer grasses stood tall and golden amid drab fallen weeds. The thorny canes of wild berries arced down in a tangle to the frozen ground. Warily, I edged by them, not wanting to get my clothing torn. Finally, I took a last look over my shoulder up the hill. It was time to get back on the road. I stepped out of the trees that edged the asphalt—and slipped on the leaves in the shallow ditch so that I lay flat on my back. Within a few seconds, I knew that I was unhurt; my thick layers of winter clothing had padded my fall—and the fall itself had put me in an unusual position. Like a spelunker who ventures down a shaft and discovers that it opens into a high-ceilinged cavern, I looked up in wonder at the sky, which was intersected by the dark tree branches like the leading that frames a stained-glass window. Grateful for the moment's rest and the glimpse of beauty, I righted myself, dusted the leaves off my coat, and headed home.

SUMMARY

Gratitude is at the center of the Reiki principles. Like the human heart, which pumps lifeblood throughout the physical body, gratitude sustains our spiritual lives. Like the heart chakra, with its ability to transmute negative into positive through the power of unconditional love, gratitude transforms negative thinking into an attitude of appreciation, positive well-being, and hope.

Gratitude offers shelter and sanctuary for the soul. In gratitude, we can rest from all the activities and conversations of the day, and all the problems and crises. In gratitude, we can be at home with Spirit. We can sit at a table and give thanks, both for gifts already received and those we're about to receive. When we allow ourselves to partake of this feast of blessings, we feel spiritually replenished and renewed. Gratitude assures us that we are loved, protected, and provided for—and allows us to leave only when we've been restored to a state of grace.

Gratitude can make beautiful stepping-stones out of whatever troubles arise on our way. Although we may face genuine obstacles, gratitude helps us regain a positive outlook so that we can problem-solve rather than engage in self-pity, and find support rather than retreat in helplessness and despair. When we feel grateful despite difficulties, we inspire others as well, who share their own stories with us, offering hope and the healing of friendship and community.

It's a pleasure to contemplate the pattern of a life lived with appreciation for its challenges as well as its opportunities, for its demands and obligations as well as its moments of ease. In gratitude, we breathe in the glory of the day, accept our own place in the world as right, experience the pleasure of our senses, and recognize our inner guidance as the compass of the soul. When we invite gratitude into our lives like a welcome guest, it brings along good company: well-being; a sense of possibility, opportunity, and hope; contentment; connection; happy expectations—and joy.

Joy is the final gift of gratitude. It can muscle in on any pity party, if we let it;

it can open a closed heart; it can invite the reluctant traveler gently forward, for just around the next bend, in just a moment, there will be something interesting and worthwhile to experience or someone whose company we will treasure.

MORE SUGGESTIONS FOR PRACTICE

✤ Practice Reiki with gratitude for the perception of the energy that flows through your hands, and for the healing you and your client receive. At the end of any hands-on or distant-healing session, make it a point to thank your client for being willing to receive Reiki.

✤ Recite the Reiki principles morning and night, just as Mikao Usui recommended, or if you prefer, say them silently to yourself before you do Reiki each day. Repetition will help anchor the suggestion to "be grateful" in the conscious and subconscious levels of your mind, making it easier to live in gratitude.

✤ Allow your recitation of the Reiki principles to inspire you to practice the spiritual discipline of mindfulness. Be present to each moment of your experience so you can acknowledge and appreciate all that is good. Let gratitude suffuse your life like a sweet scent so that you feel always on the verge of contentment and delight.

✤ Go one step further than reciting the Reiki principles by doing a brief meditation. Standing, sitting, or kneeling in a comfortable posture, focus on your breathing. Deliberately slow it down. Let yourself relax. Appreciate your quiet mind. Then open your awareness to thoughts and feelings of gratitude. Your car is back from the shop and working well. Good. Your rose bush has just started to bloom. Good. Your alarm clock radio played a song you liked this morning. Good. Gently, without any struggle, allow quiet thoughts of gratitude to open your heart. Meditate in this way for five or ten minutes (whatever length of time feels right to you), then take this awareness and appreciation of the good in your life with you into your day.

✤ A friend says, "Like attracts like. When I feel grateful, I attract more good into my life so that I have even more for which to feel grateful." Make up your own affirmation of gratitude and its power in your life using the present tense, the first-person viewpoint, and positive language. Write your affirmation on pieces of sticky-backed paper and fasten them to your alarm clock and your bathroom mirror, to the wall plug by the coffeepot, and on your car's dashboard. Throughout the day, recite the affirmation to yourself often.

❧ When you're sick, do Reiki—and practice gratitude by thanking your body for every tiny improvement in the quality of your health. In one of her early books, Sark, author of *Sark's New Creative Companion: Ways to Free Your Creative Spirit,* tells an inspiring story of a woman who survived a car accident only to be told by her doctors that she would never walk again. Instead, she thanked her physical body, especially her toes, feet, and legs, for every sensation that returned—and made a complete recovery.

❧ Use your Reiki-charged hands above your dinner plate to make your food more healthy and nourishing. Be grateful that you have the ability to bless your food with energy.

❧ If you enjoy prayer, say grace before meals. Use whatever prayer you were taught as a child or learn how people of other religions and cultures say grace. The book, *The Bridge of Stars: 365 Prayers, Blessings, and Meditations from Around the World,* offers many wonderful possibilities.

❧ Write thank-you notes. Not only does this practice exemplify good, old-fashioned manners, but it will warm your heart to reflect on others' kindness, make them feel valued, and strengthen the bonds of friendship. Yes, you can call or e-mail with the same results, but actually writing a note requires a physical effort and a commitment of time and energy that takes you deeper into the experience of gratitude.

❧ Say "thank you" to strangers for a smile, to cashiers as they complete your purchase, to gas-station attendants for manning the pumps in the cold, to your minister for a good sermon, to your child's teacher for caring enough to write a note about his or her progress, to those who expect thanks, and to those who don't expect it. Extend this practice to include family members from whom you have inherited a character trait or learned something useful. Extend it even farther to include members of your spiritual family—your Reiki ancestors, beginning with Mikao Usui.

✤ Practice gratitude for your own life, for your physical body, and for your senses, which enable you to experience this world, whether or not they're fully functioning. Be glad you can appreciate the dazzling blue of an October sky, even if you don't have 20-20 vision; that you can hear the quiet hum of traffic, even if you need a hearing aid; that you can savor the scent and taste of honey-sweetened tea; and enjoy the slight weight of a pen between your fingers as you write. Enjoying your senses is a way to celebrate your own vitality.

✤ Keep a gratitude journal. Sarah Ban Breathnach, author of *Simple Abundance: A Daybook of Comfort and Joy,* recommends writing down a minimum of five things for which you feel grateful at the end of each day. Of course, you can write more! She recommends this process as transforming.[3]

✤ Fall asleep at night doing hands-on Reiki on your heart or abdomen. Instead of reviewing your to-do list for tomorrow, count your blessings—and sleep peacefully and well.

6

INTEGRITY

"Do an Honest Day's Work"

In English, the fourth Reiki principle is most commonly translated as a recommendation to "do an honest day's work." This encouragement to work with integrity is, perhaps, only half the story: Frank Arjava Petter has offered two translations that hint at a fuller, richer meaning. In *Reiki Fire: New Information about the Origins of the Reiki Power; A Complete Manual,* he uses this wording: "Work hard today (meditative practice)."[1] The following year, in *Reiki: The Legacy of Dr. Usui,* he provides a slightly different translation: "Work hard (on yourself)."[2]

The word *integrity* may be defined as the quality or trait of rigorous adherence to the highest professional standards or moral, ethical, or spiritual values. Yet there's another definition that bears consideration here. In its earliest meaning—and one it still retains—the word *integrity* means "wholeness." The fourth Reiki principle may be understood as inviting us to do our best, whatever our occupation. However, the alternate translations hint that to do our best, we must know ourselves and work hard to become whole—healthy in body and mind, heart and soul.

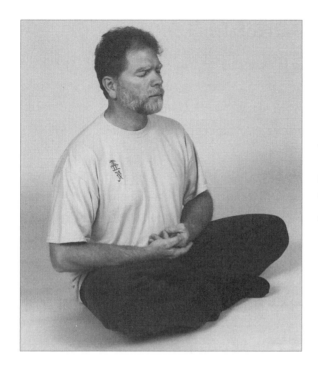

The fourth principle encourages us to look within to learn more about our essential nature.

This makes wonderful sense. Reiki healing is holistic, bringing healing on all levels. Since the example of Mikao Usui's life and the recommendations recorded on the Usui Memorial encourage us to begin to practice Reiki on ourselves, we can understand the reinforcement to continually work on our own healing implicit in the fourth principle. When we're willing to do this work on ourselves, to address any remaining issues that need healing each day, not only does our health and well-being greatly improve, but we also gain a sense of both partnership and union with Source or Spirit. This alliance with the energy instructs us in some of the qualities of our essential nature—peace, serenity, gratitude, kindness, and integrity, in its many senses—wholeness or soundness, the capacity for moral courage, the discipline to strive for creative excellence, and the willingness to act in accordance with our highest nature. The fourth principle, which seems to invite us to work to the standards of the external world, at the same time, encourages us to look within. Not only through Reiki self-treatment and client practice but also through meditation, contemplation, and reflection we learn about our true nature. Our consciousness of our connection to Spirit influences our work. Whatever we do in the world is elevated to a higher level and made healing by the energy that flows through us and our hands.

REIKI TEACHES INTEGRITY

The practice of Reiki hands-on healing teaches us that Reiki relieves pain, stanches the flow of blood, and accelerates healing. It helps us become whole and well again, restored to physical balance, mental calm, and emotional stability. We learn this through the results of treatment after treatment on ourselves and others.

Yet each treatment teaches us about wholeness in another way: each time we place our Reiki-charged hands over our eyes, heart, or abdomen, we're gently invited to think about our relationship with the Source of this healing flow. What does it mean to be a channel for healing energy? If Reiki enhances a natural ability to bring healing, is every human being already connected to the Source of healing? As we learn to trust that the energy will always be there for us to bring healing whenever we need it and whenever we want to offer it to others, we come into a deeper understanding of our relationship to Source—and we are invited to reflect on wholeness even more deeply. What does it mean to be at "one with Spirit"? What does it mean to be able to radiate the Reiki energy all day, every day—one of the goals that Japanese practitioners set for themselves? Is it possible to live our ordinary lives with a constant, gentle awareness of Spirit? Does Reiki help us to heal on all levels so that we may experience the wholeness of our human nature and our union with the divine?

Consider also the lessons of Reiki distant healing: once attuned at this level, even without personal knowledge of a client, we can send healing energy that is effective in bringing relief from pain and comfort from distress; and it doesn't matter if the client is in a location we've never visited. The wonderful, mysterious energy of Reiki can span the distance and precisely locate the client, with just a bit of information from us: identification of the client by name or a clear visualization and expression of the intention to offer healing. How is this possible? The success of Reiki distant healing implies an energetic infrastructure that spans the globe and connects every individual consciousness to every other individual consciousness. We are one in Spirit. Coming to accept this truth about our essential nature allows us to embrace our unity with Spirit and with all of life.

NOW YOU:
EXPLORE SACRED GROUND

Reiki distant healing occurs in the energy, in sacred space and time, unlimited by our concepts of political borders or chronological division into past, present, and future. If you're a Reiki II practitioner, you may feel quite content to send Reiki to a friend in the hospital across town; it brings healing and comfort to your friend, and eases your mind and heart to be able to offer this blessing, even when you're unable to visit the hospital. This is the most common way to use the distant-healing method: to send Reiki to someone who is absent or at a geographic distance.

However, once you have gained an easy familiarity with the distant-healing method you were taught, you might like to experiment with learning more about the effectiveness of Reiki sent across time. The results are sometimes mind boggling! To give the experiment a fair chance of success, try doing it every day over a period of, say, ten days or one month. Early each morning, send Reiki forward in time to yourself. After calling yourself in as a client, you might use this wording: "I offer you Reiki healing forward in time to be received, as needed, throughout the day." Remind yourself that you have free will to accept or reject the healing offered, release the outcome, and draw the symbols you were taught. Then see what it feels like to walk into the energy as you go about your day. Just as you feel yourself losing your train of thought in mid-sentence at an important meeting, you'll recover the thought and remember the point you must make; or just before a reckless driver goes careening down the street toward where you stand, you'll be guided to step back to safety, out of the racing car's way. At such moments you may notice the energy as if it were a shimmering curtain or a tingling in the air you breathe and move in. This is startling, beautiful, and healing—and it reveals Reiki's willingness to support you wherever you are, whatever the time of day, and whatever you are doing.

Is it right to talk about Reiki's "willingness"? Is this anthropomorphizing at its best—or worst? Whenever we do Reiki and witness healing that is beyond the scope of human intelligence and training, we are invited to contemplate the Source of that healing and recognize that its intelligence far exceeds our own; often, the energy's "willingness" to bring healing overcomes our own conscious misgivings and the client's loss of hope. When we do Reiki, we have the opportunity to come to know the Source of Spirit-guided life-force energy. Although it may be years before we feel comfortable acknowledging a higher power that guides the healing that occurs as we do Reiki, in time, we may decide, as Hawayo Takata did, "Reiki power—God power," or as Reiki Master Beth Gray often said to her students, "Reiki is the power of unconditional love." Whatever Reiki is, however we choose to think of it, it's worthwhile to come into a more conscious awareness of our relationship to the energy and to contemplate each experience we have as a revelation of its nature. Each experience teaches us more about union with Spirit and the wholeness of consciousness.

THE HONOR OF CHUJIRO HAYASHI

Most Reiki practitioners and teachers are acquainted with the single photograph of Dr. Chujiro Hayashi that is in the public domain. The image is of his face only: a dynamic young man smiles at us, his dark eyes shining with confidence and happiness. Surely, we think, he must have had an amazing sense of humor, a loving heart, and an open-minded nature. He seems so joyful! He must have delighted in Reiki.

Chujiro Hayashi (1879–1940) was a physician by training and an officer in the Japanese Navy who rose to the rank of captain before retiring. A family man with a wife and children, he was one of Mikao Usui's closest followers.[3] Yet we know far less about him than we know about Hawayo Takata, his first Western student. This is, in part, because Takata's story of the early history of Reiki focused largely on Mikao Usui. However, she did share some stories of her relationship with Hayashi with some of her Reiki master students, who have passed them along. In particular, she recalled his visit to Hawaii to lecture on Reiki and to certify her, and she also told the story of his death.

When Hiroshi Doi first visited the West and began to share information about Reiki's origins, Reiki masters here were surprised that Hayashi seemed to have so little place in the historical accounts. After Usui's death, two retired admirals who had served in the Japanese Navy presided over the Usui Reiki Ryoho Gakkai, the learning society established during Usui's time to continue the teaching of Reiki. Hayashi, who had such an important role in Takata's life, was strangely absent from the ranks of chairpersons. Additional research confirmed that he had directed a Reiki clinic in Tokyo, the same one where Takata had received treatment for her medical condition and was cured. This clinic had been established during Usui's lifetime. Now Reiki historians believe that Hayashi established the clinic and maintained it as a separate center of Reiki instruction at Usui's specific instruction.

Hayashi is also thought to have worked with Usui to develop the attunement process to enable a teacher to quickly pass on the ability to do Reiki healing; Usui's earliest students were probably attuned to the energy simply through his intention and presence. Such "attunements" may have taken only moments—or days, weeks, or months in the presence of the founder. As more and more people became interested in learning Reiki, it became impractical for Usui to give attunements in this way. Instead, he sat with his students in meditation, recited or sang a poem, and then led them in reciting the Reiki principles. The energy was transferred to them as he willed, through this very gentle process. The development of an even more rapid attunement process probably occurred toward the end of Usui's life, at the request of some of those he had initiated as teachers. After Usui's death, Hayashi, working separately from the Gakkai, continued to develop and refine the attunement process at his clinic and teaching center.[4]

As a result of Usui's instruction that Hayashi establish and maintain a Reiki clinic in Tokyo and teach from that location, the use of Reiki for physical healing as the foundation of health, well-being, and happiness became Hayashi's strong focus. Today, in a traditional beginner Reiki class taught by one of the spiritual descendants of Hayashi and Takata, this emphasis remains even though Reiki is acknowledged to be a source of healing on all levels. As a result, as Mr. Doi has said, "In the West, you have many miracles."[5] In Japan, within the Gakkai, greater emphasis has been placed on using Reiki for spiritual healing. Now it is the privilege of Reiki practitioners and teachers worldwide to be able to study both traditions and work toward health, well-being, and happiness by using techniques from both traditions.

So we must acknowledge Chujiro Hayashi's great contribution to the lives of Reiki practitioners and teachers worldwide. Yet in class, most Reiki masters shy away from telling the story of his death. We speak of his importance in the life of Hawayo Takata, as the physician who cured her with Reiki and taught her to the master level, giving her permission to teach in the West, but we avoid mentioning that Hayashi took his own life to avoid being recalled to active duty in the Japanese Navy before the start of the Second World War.

"What do you mean? How could he take his own life?" students want to know. "Did he fall on a knife in a ritual suicide?"

It seems too sad a loss and too incomprehensible a choice for most Reiki masters to say more. Often, however, the reason they don't say more is that they do not know the story of his death. They lack the details. So here is a brief retelling:

One night early in 1940, Hawayo Takata dreamed of her teacher, Chujiro Hayashi, wearing a white silk kimono, and pacing back and forth. The dream was unsettling, and on waking, she felt an urgency to see him. She booked passage to Japan, where she went to visit the Hayashi family. She saw with her own eyes that her teacher was well. However, Mrs. Hayashi informed her that he would be making his "transition" before Japan and the United States went to war. He was certain that if he did not, he would be recalled to active duty as an officer in the Imperial Japanese Navy and made to be responsible for much loss of life. As a Buddhist and Reiki master, this was completely unacceptable to him, for it violated his highest spiritual values. He could not and would not live such a life.

So he came to accept the necessity of his transition, which would be a gentle departure from his physical body into eternal life—for he believed that life does not end—but he did not yet know the exact date and time. He told Takata to go south to visit Kyoto, Japan, and to study healing methods used in the spas there until he sent for her. In early May 1940, Takata received the telegram from the Hayashis asking for her to return. She took a night train and arrived in the very early morning; the Hayashis invited her to join them at breakfast, and talked and laughed with her as if nothing were wrong.

This made Takata wonder what was going on and what the "transition" would mean. After breakfast, Hayashi talked to Takata for some time about

154

the disposition of his property and the future of the Reiki clinic in Tokyo. Then, in late morning, other family members and friends began to arrive for a buffet lunch. Hayashi dressed in a ceremonial white silk robe to share this last meal with his guests. After the meal, he thanked his guests for coming and told them he would make his transition very soon: an artery would rupture, to be quickly followed by another and another, and he would feel no pain. Even as he spoke, the process had already begun. He had lived a life of peace, and he reassured them that this passage would also be peaceful. Life does not end, so there is no need for tears or sorrow. In this way, he encouraged his guests to continue their celebration of his life, for they had gathered to honor him.

Just as he had predicted, these events occurred. With the rupturing of the third artery, Hayashi fell backward into his wife's waiting arms. His body was taken to Tokyo, for viewing by those who wished to pay their respects. These included many Reiki students and patients who had been taught and healed at the Reiki clinic he had established at Usui's request. Then his body was cremated and a Zen Buddhist funeral ceremony performed.

This retelling is based on three sources: my memory of Beth Gray's recounting of this story at a few of the Reiki I classes at which I assisted (she did not always tell this story); *Living Reiki: Takata's Teachings*, by Takata-trained Reiki Master Fran Brown;[6] and *Reiki: Hawayo Takata's Story*, by another of Takata's students, Helen J. Haberly.[7]

In Fran Brown's account is a fascinating comment regarding Hayashi's final instructions to Takata: "He instructed her to leave Japan and return to her home, and told her in which places she would be safe during the war. He also told her what the outcome of the war would be. As with many people who practice Reiki, he had learned to trust the messages given to him through his own intuition."[8]

Hayashi's appreciation of his intuition offers a clue to anyone who wishes to have a deeper understanding of Hayashi's death. Over many years of practice, he was guided through his meditations and use of Reiki to understand and value intuitive impressions that arose on the flow of the energy. Perhaps his decision to make his transition at a particular time and date was a guided one. As for the method of his physical death, how could he have accomplished this? Was he responsible for this occurrence, or did Spirit accomplish this with Hayashi's freewill consent? Or did he surrender his dilemma to Spirit and receive foreknowledge of its resolution through his meditations and practice of Reiki?

Probably, we shall never know the answers to these questions. However, we can honor Hayashi's choice as one of great integrity, instead of avoiding the subject. Hayashi, a vital, healthy man of sixty-two, made the decision to leave his physical body rather than become involved in war, a decision which must have taken extraordinary courage. How deeply he must have valued his spiritual life, and how committed he must have been to embodying the Reiki principles. Let us be inspired by his sacrifice to live our lives with integrity.*

BEING THE
LIGHT IN THE DARKNESS

When Charlie Wagg retired as a policeman, getting another job wasn't a priority for him. Instead, he looked forward to relaxing at home and doing lots of Reiki. Yet in fall 1999, when an opening came up in the county sheriff's department for a deputy sheriff in the courts division, he applied for the job and was immediately hired. Since then, he has worked full-time as a county deputy sheriff, providing courtroom security and transporting prisoners back and forth to the courthouse from prisons and detention centers across the county. He also works in the D.A.R.E. program, educating schoolchildren about the dangers of drug and alcohol abuse.

At first, he had some misgivings about the job. If anything, it put him into even closer contact with people who were in trouble with the law and intensely angry at the legal and judicial system that had placed them behind bars. Then Charlie realized that hiding behind the sullen faces and the insolent attitudes

---

*Dr. Chujiro Hayashi chose to make his transition because he faced an exceptional circumstance. He took no physical action to end his life, but was guided by Spirit to be prepared for the event and was granted foreknowledge of the day and the hour. Suicide is not being condoned here as a solution to life's problems. If you are seriously depressed and suffering from suicidal thoughts, see a mental health professional immediately to receive counseling. Use Reiki as complementary therapy to calm your emotions and mind.

were people struggling with deep disappointments, depression, and fear. They were, in fact, in great need of support and healing.

So Charlie began to rethink his plans for retirement. Maybe he was working in exactly the right place. Maybe he was fulfilling his soul's purpose. Meanwhile, he continued to practice Reiki and learn more about its early history. When he discovered that one of Mikao Usui's early occupations, before his work with Reiki, had been as a prison warden, Charlie thought of this as validation of his choice. He began to look for ways to bring Reiki "on the job." Primarily, he hoped to show by example how to live a good life—to offer kindness, honesty, appreciation, calm strength, and peace.

However, he found that he could do even more than lead by example. At times, he could make subtle use of Reiki to help the prisoners in his care. On one occasion, he was ordered to escort a juvenile male prisoner to and from the courtroom so that he could enter a guilty plea before the judge. Charlie observed that as the district attorney questioned the prisoner, the young man became more and more upset. His parents were present at the hearing, and he was pale and perspiring, clearly nervous about going over the details of his crime. Discreetly, Charlie raised his hands to beam Reiki to the prisoner on the stand. The flow was intense, and the prisoner responded almost immediately, becoming calmer and more composed, his voice quiet and steady. Charlie continued to send Reiki to the young man for the remainder of his court appearance.

On another occasion, Charlie was asked to escort an adult male prisoner back to the detention center after a brief courtroom proceeding. He was warned that this prisoner had paranoid schizophrenia and could become violent if upset. As Charlie approached the man in the hallway outside the courtroom, he saw that the prisoner was already agitated. As he handcuffed the prisoner, he felt Reiki radiating intensely to the man. Immediately, the prisoner became calmer. Another officer commented, "Charlie, I don't know what you're doing, but you stay with that prisoner. Whatever it is, it's working!" Charlie felt pleased that he could help the prisoner with Reiki and that it had such an immediate, beneficial effect.

Now when Charlie talks about his work as a deputy sheriff, he does so with a sense of pride. It's not what he expected or envisioned he would do in retirement, but he's confident that it is the right work for him to do at this time. It satisfies his desire to be a Reiki healer and accords with his soul's purpose.

NOW YOU:
AN HONEST DAY'S WORK

How do we demonstrate integrity on the job? Although being honest, dependable, productive, and committed to quality goes a long way toward achieving this goal, for a Reiki practitioner, integrity on the job can mean something more. Whatever our occupation, we have the opportunity to embody the values of the Reiki principles in the workplace.

One way to be kind on the job is to offer to do Reiki informally to relieve a tension headache, tight shoulders, or tired eyes. However, most of us don't feel comfortable being so direct in presenting Reiki to colleagues. Instead, we must *be* Reiki: peaceful, calm, appreciative, honest and dependable, and kind. When we behave in this way, we bring light into the workplace: the atmosphere improves, everyone feels more positive and upbeat, people are inspired

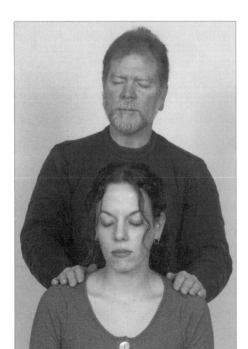

Reiki can be offered informally in the workplace.

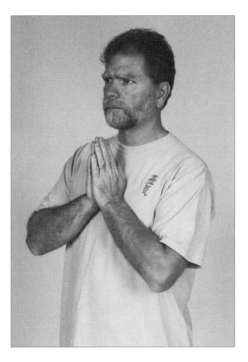

Commitment to reciting the Reiki principles at the start of the day can make it easier to remember them in the workplace.

to do their best—and we feel good about our work and about ourselves. This is a wonderful way to bring healing.

What can you do on the job to *be* Reiki? Take some time to think about your on-the-job behaviors and how you might want to modify them. If you feel as though you tend to forget about Reiki during the business day, you might want to get up a few minutes earlier to recite the Reiki principles and do some hands-on healing. If you're an advanced practitioner, you might even send Reiki forward in time to yourself and to your coworkers to be received as needed throughout the day to support health and well-being.

During the workday, if you feel pushed or pressured, you may find it hard to maintain the calm frame of mind that comes from doing Reiki. Write the Reiki principles on a piece of sticky-backed paper to attach to your office wall or desk surface where you will often see them. When you feel that you're losing your temper, composure, or sense of control, reread the words to steady your commitment to embody the principles. This brief action resets your intention to stay on spiritual track, which can help you achieve and maintain integrity.

AT A REIKI PRINCIPLES WORKSHOP:
EXPLORING INTEGRITY

In summer 2007, my friend Reiki Master Ellen Philips and I began to teach a workshop for practitioners and teachers interested in deepening their understanding of the Reiki principles. The workshop quickly evolved from a one-day to two-day format so we would have more time to consider each of the principles individually and to offer more meditations and exercises for healing. The greatest surprise of the class was the power of the Reiki energy. As we explored the principles one by one, more and more energy poured into the room, which we absorbed as healing. In short order, we all felt good and happy.

Yet our discussions were often quite serious, particularly regarding integrity. To begin our discussion, we did a journal exercise. "I'm going to ask you a few questions," I told the class "that I want you to pose to yourself. You can easily answer all the questions in more than one way. In your notebook, I would like you to write down your first thoughts, the first half a dozen words that pop into your mind in reply. When you've had the chance to jot these down, I'll ask you the next question. Are you ready?"

Everyone nodded, pens poised above blank pages.

"This is the first question that I want you to ask yourself: 'Who am I?'" I waited as the practitioners wrote.

When I had everyone's attention again, I invited the students to respond to the next question: "What is my soul's purpose?" Again, they jotted down their first thoughts.

One by one, I raised more questions, pausing after each one for a few quiet minutes to allow the students to record their thoughts: What is my passion? What are my strengths? What are my weaknesses? What is my heart's desire? Some of the questions required clarification. One student asked, "Is pursuing your passion the same as satisfying your heart's desire?"

"No, I don't think so," I said. "Our passions are individual. One of you might love gardening, another creative writing, another jewelry making. You can pursue those on your own and enjoy them all your lives. Satisfying your heart's desire may require a lot more work! Let me pose the question in another way: what would it take for you to feel completely happy and whole, completely in love with your life right now?"

The students lowered their heads, eyes focused on the moving pen on the page and the next word they would reveal to themselves.

After the students had responded to all six questions, I asked them to share with the class the single answer that seemed most true for them to each of the questions in turn. They had replied to the question, "Who am I?" with amazing wisdom: "I am a spark of divine light," "I am a child of God," "I am a manifestation of divine consciousness," "I am a spiritual being in a physical body enjoying the journey of a lifetime." Their responses to the questions that had followed were more personally revealing. Someone acknowledged a love of traveling, another felt blessed with strong willpower, and one admitted to a habit of procrastination.

The final question, "What is your heart's desire?" generated a lot of discussion. One Reiki master, a widow in her forties, was convinced that she could only be happy if she could find a man who would love and marry her.

"That's a problem," I told her. "I hope that you do find your soul mate and can achieve wedded bliss, but what if you don't? Are you willing to delay happiness for the rest of your life just because he's not around?"

"Well, I just know that I will feel happier when he's in my life," she said, fidgeting in her chair.

"You very well may," I agreed, "but please don't postpone happiness. Open up to the possibility that you can feel happy today. Claim it."

She pursed her lips, as if considering.

"Look," I told her, "when I did this exercise with you, I wrote down something similar for my heart's desire, but my guess is that the gentleman I hope to meet is probably herding sheep on a mountain in Scotland."

Ellen, my co-teacher, interrupted. "Wearing a kilt?"

"I expect so," I said, "and playing the bagpipes." We all laughed. I returned to my point: "So as long as he's there, and I'm here, I'm going to claim as much happiness as I can without him. I'm not waiting. I want to live a good life and feel as much contentment, as much peace, as much joy as I can right *now*. That's part of the reason for this workshop: the practice of Reiki and the Reiki principles offer us a secret method of inviting happiness. It's possible for us *now*. Do you really want to postpone it?"

She relented with a smile. "Okay," she said, "I get it."

However, the exercise wasn't quite finished. There was one more question that I wanted the Reiki practitioners and teachers in the class to ask themselves: "If you never achieve your heart's desire, can you still commit to doing your best today and every day that follows? To put it another way, if your vision of fulfillment never manifests, can you live with integrity anyway?"

They listened, sitting back in their chairs, thinking about the implications. There were only two possible answers. A clear "yes" reflected self-knowledge and commitment to the soul's purpose, while a "no" signaled a need for further self-exploration and some healing. The commitment to live with integrity requires wholeness, and it can only be made with surety by someone who wishes that self-respect to remain unassailable. The commitment cannot be allowed to waiver, despite an apparent lack of success in achieving other goals. Whatever our circumstances, whatever crises we face, we need to live by our own highest values in order to stay on course for health, well-being, and happiness. Integrity is the light within us, allowed to shine. It illuminates the path we travel like a miner's headlamp, even when we travel through darkness. It is wise never to set integrity aside. It shows us the way ahead, sometimes one step at a time. It keeps us on safe ground.

NOW YOU:
FIND YOUR WAY TO WHOLENESS

You may easily adapt this workshop exercise for your own use. Find a quiet, comfortable corner where you won't be interrupted for forty-five minutes to an hour. In a notebook, answer the following questions, in the order presented here, taking five minutes or so to respond to each one. Jot down your first thoughts quickly, indicating your reply with a word or phrase. Allow yourself to generate at least a half-dozen answers to each question; the more responses you have, the more likely you are to get beneath the surface of conscious thought and reveal something of your true nature to yourself.

Who am I?

What is my purpose?

What is my passion?

What are my strengths?

What are my weaknesses?

What is my heart's desire?

If I never achieve my heart's desire, will I do my best anyway?

Try not to anticipate the next question. Be fully present in the moment as you reply to each one. In this way, the exercise becomes a kind of meditation as well as a tool for greater self-knowledge. There are no wrong answers. However, the pattern of your answers may help you identify your priorities, not as you think they are, but as you actually live them throughout the day. For example, if you answer the question, "Who am I?" once with "watercolor artist" and a dozen times with phrases that reference your role as a husband and father, you'll have a vivid illustration of your lived priorities, as well as a clue to your creative nature and ambitions.

The questions, "What are my strengths?" and "What are my weaknesses?" may also invite you to separate professional standards and social expectations from your sense of self-worth. Filtering through your replies will help you see how accountable you are to others and to yourself. If there's a discrepancy, you may want to consider the reasons and think about how you might achieve a better balance. Your replies may also help you identify your highest values. If you aren't already living by these values, you may want to shift your behavior slightly now in their direction—making a gentle course correction—so that your life feels more on track.

Learning more about your weaknesses may show you something about yourself that needs healing. For example, if you admit that you're disorganized, you can focus on healing that quality in yourself through Reiki distant healing. You may also want to reflect on your relationship with yourself in light of the Reiki principles. When you call yourself disorganized, are you being realistic or self-critical and unkind? Is the way to heal this issue better household and time management, or is it appropriate to relax your perfectionist standards? Other questions that may lead you into a greater awareness of your own need for emotional and mental healing are these: What do I dislike doing? What tasks do I put off? Whom do I dislike? Whom do I avoid? Where do I resist going? The answers to these questions are clues to patterns of avoidance and denial.

For some practitioners, this exercise in self-awareness may bring up painful memories and uncomfortable realizations. If we have been dishonest with others or ourselves in the past, we may find the challenge of reclaiming integrity almost overwhelming. Yet if we are to enjoy wholeness and well-being, we must accept the challenge. Just for today, now, in this moment, we can make the effort to be truthful with others and ourselves. We can keep our promises and honor our commitments. We can be reliable on the job and dependable at home. This may demand of us an almost microscopic focus on the present moment. The emotional baggage of the past must be set down and hope for the future postponed. All our personal energy and attention must be wholly given to behaving with integrity *now*. Only then does reclaiming lost integrity and healing damaged self-respect become a manageable task.

In private, we can also send Reiki back in time to free ourselves from any burden of guilt and shame over past wrongdoing that we have carried forward into the present. This will help free us to behave with integrity today. In addition, we can send Reiki forward in time to help ourselves remain true to the spiritual values that we want to embody now in our lives. Through this effort, we may gradually come to realize that there's more that we want to do to make amends for wrongdoing than simply send healing into the past and live with integrity in the present. If this recognition occurs, meditation and prayer may help us become clear on how to proceed.

Being aware of the ways in which we still need healing on all levels can help us determine how to direct Reiki to ourselves as clients when we do distant healing; we may offer Reiki to heal damaged self-esteem, self-sabotaging behaviors, or an inability to forgive. With increased self-awareness and Reiki focused on emotional and mental healing, we may take the next steps forward in our lives with greater confidence, optimism, and trust in ourselves. Our spiritual values become an inner moral compass, enabling us to proceed with a sense of clear direction. As we integrate the necessary healing and live with greater integrity, we discover that we are enjoying our lives with a whole heart.

INTEGRITY
AND FULFILLMENT

On the way to becoming whole and happy, many Reiki practitioners and teachers find themselves reflecting on their unrealized dreams and undeveloped talents:

I always wanted to take up photography, a practitioner thinks as he passes a display of camera equipment in a store. *I wonder if I would feel comfortable using one of those new digital cameras. They don't look all that complicated, and I really like the idea of being able to edit the shots before ever printing them.*

On an errand into a shopping center, another practitioner stops into a craft shop and wanders through the aisles until she finds herself stopped before shelves of yarns. She cannot help but touch the soft skeins of thread and admire the subtle colors. She thinks she might enjoy learning to knit, if she could find an introductory class.

"I've always had this crazy ambition to learn to fly an airplane," a Reiki master confides to his fellow passenger on a commuter shuttle between Boston and New York. "I've thought about it on and off since I was a kid, and I start to think about it all over again every time I fly. I can't seem to get the idea out of my head."

No matter what the forgotten dream or the "crazy ambition," sometimes giving it serious consideration can yield rewards. At the minimum, we gain greater insight into ourselves and develop deeper appreciation for our individuality. Beyond that, we may feel more excited about the future. The recognition that we might be able to realize some inner potential can motivate us to pursue training, develop skills, refine talents, and accomplish goals. When we allow ourselves to expand, to become more fully who we're meant to be, we span the distance between our limited "reality" and our unlimited dreams. We become more complete, fulfilled, and whole. We find that in pursuing our passions, we fall in love with our lives. We get happy!

In terms of psychology, to enjoy our lives we must fulfill both basic needs that support survival and higher needs that help us become self-actualized. When we honor our uniqueness, pursue our personal interests, and realize more of our potential, we're fulfilling these higher needs and being true to ourselves as individuals. This is another way that we can work toward living with integrity. The fourth Reiki principle invites us to "do an honest day's work" and to "work hard" on ourselves; we may strive to live with integrity to honor our spiritual nature, but we may also endeavor to lead full, happy lives that express our human nature. We are spiritual and human; to be whole, we must accept both as one.

NOW YOU:
DISCOVER A LOST DREAM
OR A LYING-IN-WAIT TALENT

Remember what you thought you would be when you grew up? When you were about six or seven, you may have imagined joining the circus and becoming a clown. A little later on, you may have decided that you wanted to be the quarterback on a pro football team or the prima ballerina in a ballet troupe. Maybe you considered becoming a translator at the United Nations or becoming a teacher of English as a second language in a foreign country. Whatever that early dream was, you probably set it aside to do something more practical; most people do.

However, all dreams provide clues about the dreamer. Make a date with yourself for some quiet time in a beautiful setting, with notebook and pen handy. Write it down as an appointment on your calendar—and keep that commitment to yourself. You might start off with a stroll through a park or a public garden, or walk by a playground where you can watch children. What attracts and holds your attention? What engages your senses most fully? Does the scuffle-bounce-thud of a pickup basketball game stop you in your tracks? Does the scent of fresh-baked bread remind you of happy hours spent in your grandmother's kitchen? Open your mind. Let the world around you remind you of what you most enjoy and what you enjoyed as a child.

When you've stretched your legs and expanded your awareness to include the broader world, find a bench, rest your eyes, remember as many of your childhood dreams as you can, and write them down. Don't judge them as absurd or unrealistic. Just recall them and write them down in a list. All you are doing is collecting some memories—and identifying points of access into your own undeveloped country. Later on, you can look over your remembered dreams to discover which ones still awake longing in you. This is your clue to your next step.

If your childhood dreams centered on being a sports hero and you're now a stockbroker, it's a sure thing that you won't ever join the NFL, but you might enjoy getting involved in after-school coaching. If you remember feeling sad about having to give up ballet lessons because you were too busy with other activities, you may find that you get a lot of satisfaction out of an adult dance class. If everyone in your family discouraged you from becoming a circus clown, you'll be pleased to learn that clown schools exist and even part-time clowns can play center stage at children's parties, bringing laughter and smiles.

Recovering your childhood dreams and pursuing them can help the broken inner child become whole or the healthy adult fall in love with life. Discovering your own hidden talents and developing them can add new dimensions to your personality, round out your résumé, and connect you to people you would never otherwise meet: a local playwright or poet; the members of an artists' co-op or biking club; other comic book aficionados. (To find others with like interests, check out www.meetup.com. This is also a way to find other Reiki practitioners in your area.)

When we become whole, we become more engaged with life. This may be expressed through a more vibrant sense of individuality, or as commitment to community, or in a stronger connection to Spirit—or all of these. When we become whole and live with integrity, we are likely to feel in greater harmony with our world.

AN UNFORESEEN REWARD

Perhaps it shouldn't be surprising that when we attempt to live with integrity, to navigate the journey of our lives by using an inner compass that points to our highest spiritual values, we're sometimes rewarded with inspiration and guidance. This was demonstrated to me during the writing of this book.

One day, after doing Reiki, I sat at my laptop writing and rewriting for several hours. Then I decided to do some errands in my car, while there was still a bit of light left that winter afternoon. Even though my errands were just necessary chores, like going to the bank and the grocery store, I still felt that I was very much with the Reiki energy. The day felt holy, as if sanctified in some way, and I felt a sense of reverence for Spirit.

On the way home, as I drove past strip malls toward an intersection where I usually turn onto a highway, I heard an inner voice gently suggest: "Go that way. There's something for you to see." I considered the message. I had more work to do. Could I really afford to delay my arrival by even an extra half hour? The voice repeated, "Go that way. There's something for you to see." Accompanying the words, I felt a curious tugging. I heard the voice one more time, just as I was about to make my turn, and heeded it. Clicking off my turn signal, I went straight onto the unfamiliar country road.

Within a mile or so, I noticed a herd of animals dotting the hillside. There were so many that I thought they must be cows. I slowed down to get a closer look, then realized with a rush of pleasure that I was viewing an enormous herd of deer, their dull winter coats making them hard to see against the drab fields. Finally, I pulled over onto the shoulder, stopped the car, got out, and started counting . . . and counting . . . and counting. There were so many! Remembering that I had binoculars in the car, I dug them out and counted again. All along the hillside, across the patchwork blanket of a half-dozen farmers' fields, a herd of 122 deer grazed. The sight of them, so at peace and at home on the land, touched my soul.

Whenever I'm guided to find beauty or peace, to find a solution to a problem, or to see a way forward when I have felt stalled, I feel so grateful. The message reminds me that as a Reiki practitioner, I am connected to Spirit and am constantly being guided. That awareness makes me happy. This experience taught me that when I listen for that inner guidance as I do "an honest day's work," that guidance remains available to me after the work is completed, and can direct me to that which brings me support, healing, joy, and peace. As you live the values of Reiki, that guidance can do the same for you.

FOLLOWING THE ENERGY

Under a blazing midday sun, the salt marsh off the bay on the western side of Assateague Island hummed with life: Red-winged blackbirds balanced on tall stems of lush-green cordgrass, swaying a little in the warm breeze. A great blue heron posed on ungainly stilt-like legs, eyeing a mussel in the shallows. A hawk soared to a loblolly pine and perched high on a gnarled, twisted limb to watch the landscape—and to watch us.

There were five of us: four students in a Reiki master class and me. We sat on a weathered wooden bench on an observation deck off the long walkway through the salt marsh. We'd walked there in the salt air and sun to practice Reiki attunements outdoors. For the last twenty minutes, we'd seen no other park visitors. The students were eager to practice; Lauren Sage asked if she might begin.

"Yes," I said. I took my place with the other three students on the bench. Lauren stood before us, brought her hands together in gassho, closed her eyes, and bowed. For a moment, she was silent, praying. Then she circled around the bench to place her hands on my crown. She paused, and I knew that she was asking for permission to proceed. I felt her hands move again above my hand, and I heard the cries of birds and the whir of insects. I kept my eyes closed, for I had watched her do attunements many times and was confident that she needed no supervision from me. Instead, I focused my awareness on the energy, the scent of the marsh, the sounds of the birds, and the warmth of the sun on my skin.

Hearing her call my name, I opened my eyes and saw that she now stood in front of us. She had completed about half the attunement. "There's a group of tourists coming down the walkway," she said in a low voice. "They're about fifty feet away. What should I do? Should I stop?"

"No," I said, sitting back against the bench. "Lower your hands to your sides and come stand over here at the end of the bench against the railing. Everyone else, just let your hands rest in your laps, please, and keep your eyes closed."

"The attunement isn't finished," Lauren protested, as she moved to the railing.

"I know—and you're going to finish it." I was quiet for a minute, listening inwardly to the energy. "Here's what I want you to do: Close your eyes and pick up the attunement exactly where you left off. Visualize every gesture, and be just as thorough and focused as you would be if you were standing in front of us. Do you think you can do that?"

"Yes, okay. The tourists are on the observation deck now, but they seem to be staying on the other side."

"That's fine. Please, just continue the attunement as I asked."

She did so, and we all followed along, imagining each gesture and word. When she finished and said the closing prayer, we all knew the moment when the attunement was concluded. She returned to stand before us, smiling. I glanced behind her. The tourists were leaving the observation deck, walking farther along the walkway.

The students couldn't hold back their enthusiasm. "That was amazing!"

"I felt when you slapped my hands, even though you didn't slap my hands!"

"I could feel every gesture, not just for myself but for the others in line."

"Did you ever do this before?" Lauren asked me.

"No, never . . ."

"How did you know it would work?"

"I didn't know for certain, but I trust the energy. It's the energy that attunes us, and I thought that if you focused your attention, the energy would do the rest. So you did, and the energy worked through you, just not in the usual way."

"That was very powerful," one student added.

"Yes," I agreed, looking out over the rough landscape of the salt marsh. The hawk was gone from the loblolly pine, but swallows darted through the air and iridescent-winged dragonflies hovered nearby. In the distance, a band of wild horses grazed.

I felt profoundly grateful to be guided by the energy. I was reminded by that afternoon's "lesson" that when I trust what I've learned of the energy, even when I'm on unexplored ground, the energy goes forward before me and shows the way. When I am true to what I know, the energy guides me and seems to anticipate every need. The energy beckons me, inviting me to take the next step on the path of Reiki.

The more we can stay centered in the flow of the energy, the more we learn about true integrity. When we do not anger but stay anchored in the calm center of our being, we enjoy a sense of being aligned with Spirit. When we do not worry but remain serene, soothed by the energy's gentle waves radiating outward from that center, we feel more conscious of our connection to Spirit. We stay closer to our spiritual home in gratitude. We feel appreciation for the beauty and peace of our lives. Honoring our connection to Spirit, we extend honesty to others, and we're honest with ourselves. True to our essential nature, we are kind. We experience wonder and take delight in the healing blessings of Reiki. With gladness and thanks, we become aware of our own happiness.

SUMMARY

The translations of the fourth principle recommend that we do our best in the workplace and at home; they also suggest that we look inward to discover our essential nature so we can live in accordance with that nature and our highest values. By balancing our outward efforts to "do an honest day's work" with inward exploration, we can arrive at a better understanding of what within us remains to be healed. We can use Reiki energy healing and apply the Reiki principles "just for today" to support our intention to live with integrity.

Integrity is not only adherence to a high standard of behavior, but it is also the quality of wholeness or soundness. The practice of Reiki helps us to heal the past, become well in the present, and maintain health and well-being into the future. Remembrance of the Reiki principles helps us choose healthier behaviors now, so that in addition to health and well-being, we may experience greater confidence, peace of mind, and happiness.

To live with integrity requires constant vigilance: we must seek to be ever more aware of our highest spiritual values and to abide by them. This inward focus means that we are more attentive to guidance in the form of creative inspiration and intuitive impressions. These unasked-for rewards deepen our sense of connection to Spirit, which brings us comfort and joy.

MORE SUGGESTIONS
FOR PRACTICE

❧ Whenever we use distant healing, we learn a bit more about the energy's ability to be present with us, in us, and through us, and simultaneously, anywhere else in time and space. This paradox implies an energetic infrastructure—perhaps consciousness itself—that the energy can travel the way that you and I might press an elevator button for the third floor, only faster. At the speed of thought, the energy is wherever we've asked

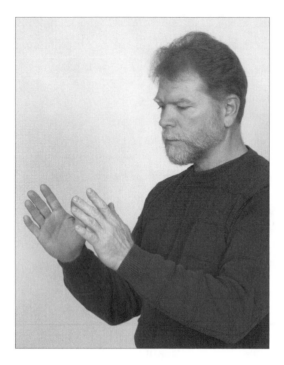

The energy can be present anywhere in space and time.

it to be, present for the purpose of healing, whether it's Leningrad; Gary, Indiana; New Orleans, Louisiana; an Earth-orbiting satellite; two o'clock tomorrow; yesterday at 5:16 p.m.; or approximately twelve years ago. The energy is unlimited in its ability to be present anywhere in space and time. Let your use of Reiki distant healing gently dissolve some of your concepts of limitation. Be inspired to claim your constant connection to Spirit, and through that connection, your connection with all other living beings. This is another way that Reiki teaches us about wholeness and integrity.

🍀 In his inspirational book *A New Earth: Awakening to Your Life's Purpose,* Eckhart Tolle writes: "In many cases, happiness is a role people play, and behind the smiling facade, there is a great deal of pain."[9] To experience real happiness, we have to be willing to recognize when we're faking the smiles just to get along with others and go on with the daily routine. While there are times when pretending we're contented and happy may seem like a good temporary solution to problems, in the long run, pretense leaves us terribly unsatisfied: we feel false and hollow, empty of integrity, disappointed in ourselves—and often, the problems still need to be resolved.

When you feel tempted to fake happiness, offer Reiki distant healing toward the situation that troubles you. If you're already many weeks, months, or years into feigning happiness, do the same kind of distant healing, but also send Reiki to yourself and to your ability to feel happiness. By playacting happiness when you're not genuinely happy, you may have diminished your capacity for joy. You can recover! Be patient, make emotional healing a priority, and commit to living "just for today" with integrity.

Integrity requires a faith in our own standards and values, and a commitment in the moment to act always in accordance with them. Sometimes this requires us to become clear on our priorities in an instant. There's a wonderful story from the Zen Buddhist tradition that illustrates this:

Two monks were walking along a path when they came to a shallow, fast-running stream. Beside the stream, a woman stood, wondering how she would get across without getting wet. The elder of the two monks offered to carry her across on his back. She gratefully accepted his kind offer and clambered onto his shoulders. They crossed the stream, with the other monk following behind. As soon as they had arrived on the opposite bank, the monk set the woman down. She thanked him and went on her way. Then the monks began to walk again along the path to their destination. An hour passed, and the younger monk asked his companion, "Why did you carry that woman across the stream? It's against the rules of our order to have any contact with women!" The older monk replied, "I set her down an hour ago. Why are *you* still carrying her?"

It's not always easy to choose between values, and sometimes we must do just that. Fortunately, the path of Reiki is experiential; that is, Reiki teaches us through our experiences, again and again. We are gently guided forward by the energy, which reveals our connection to Spirit and shows us what is "true" about our essential nature. We don't have to rely on any doctrine or dogma—not even the Reiki principles—to come to this understanding. It is important not to make the Reiki principles into a set of external rules that we follow in a soldierlike way.

Can you explore, understand, and appreciate the Reiki principles, and apply them in your life without becoming so attached to them that you use them to pass judgment on yourself or others? See if you can. Look upon the principles as helpful suggestions for bringing healing and wholeness into the present moment, but always listen to the energy that flows through your hands and the guidance from Spirit that arrives on that flow of the energy. That inner guidance is for you in the present moment. It is prior in your awareness to any words in any language, and if a choice must be made, let that guidance take precedence over the principles. What if you still feel unclear about what to do? Wait. Do Reiki. Allow the energy to relax and calm you. Be in the energy, in your own peaceful center, until you know how to proceed.

❧ When we act with integrity, we often inspire others around us to do the same. When we do our best, those who witness our efforts sometimes realize that they, too, are capable of more. Yet we live in a world that is corrupt in so many ways that we may be tempted to wonder if the commitment we make to integrity can make any difference at all. Consider the beginnings of Reiki in our time, with a single man in meditation receiving enlightenment and empowerment to bring healing. Now, a few generations later, Reiki has spread around the world; millions practice Reiki every day. Despite "appearances," please do not dismiss the value of your commitment or the impact of your efforts to act with integrity. Let your actions be like drops of pure rainwater that fall onto the surface of a lake, refreshing it and bringing it healing. Notice how the impact of your actions ripples out, and let this be a source of satisfaction and comfort to yourself and others.

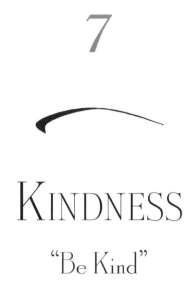

7

KINDNESS

"Be Kind"

The fifth principle is translated into English without much variation: "Be kind to all living things," "Be kind to all creatures," or most simply, "Be kind." This is an imperative that makes sense to us all on a soul level, for we understand that kindness is incendiary, a source of light and energy, both kinetic and potential. When we are kind, we allow the light within us to shine forth, to penetrate the darkness, to warm ourselves and another, and to show the way forward. We know, too, that kindness creates healing simply through human connection and the friendly offer of a helping hand. The recipient, feeling cared for, watched over, and supported, may open to receive the kindness with wonder and wordless gratitude. Saying "thank you" seems too little. Instead, the recipient remembers the kindness and looks for opportunities to be kind to others as well. Being kind is an act of spiritual revolution. It spreads the sense of caring, human kinship without words or propaganda, converting people to its cause one connection, one kindness at a time.

REIKI
TEACHES KINDNESS

The most selfless act of kindness begins in a willingness to be fully present for another in a caring way, to be sufficiently attentive to another's needs that they are acutely observed and adequately met. The Reiki energy that flows through our hands as we do hands-on or distant healing demonstrates again and again these qualities of kindness for us. Can we learn how to be kind by practicing Reiki? Yes.

Consider: whether we relax on a couch, giving Reiki to ourselves or stand table-side with our hands on a client, we gradually come to understand that the energy flows in perfect response to the need for healing. As we feel the energy radiating through our hands with steady warmth, we learn about constancy, gentleness, and comforting presence. As we ponder the various sensations we experience—a quiet hum of current, a mild tingling, or a strong pulsing vibration—we become aware of the intelligence and sensitivity with which the energy is delivered and the need for healing met. This is Spirit-guided life-force energy, channeled through our fingers and palms, accelerating healing, restoring balance, relieving pain, and sometimes working miracles. It is our task simply to be attentive to the sensations of energy. Through this practice, we realize that it is a pleasure to give loving attention to every aspect of our experience and a source of deep satisfaction to witness the process of healing. Connected, centered, grounded in the flow of the Reiki energy, we discover that it is easy to be kind.

Many people who decide to learn Reiki already value the practice of kindness before they walk in the door of their level I class. They have discovered how natural it feels to be kind and how gratifying it is to bring sincerity, warmth, and attentiveness to all their conversations and interactions with others. Often, they learn hands-on healing with a silent agenda to offer it, at the first opportunity, to a loved one who is ill or needs support. Already these individuals are adapting their work schedules to care for a sick relative at home or are sacrificing weekend hours to drive to a long-term care facility for a visit with an elderly parent. They're eager to take on any and every task that will ease the loved one's pain or difficulties. To help out, they buy the weekly groceries, tackle the bill paying, clean the kitchen, and wash the dirty dishes.

They have looked within their own hearts and made the commitment to do whatever is necessary to be present and to be kind.

Sometimes, it's this same determination to be a source of support and healing for a loved one that motivates Reiki practitioners to take the advanced course and learn distant healing. A young woman living in New York may not be able to fly home very often to be with her recently widowed mother, but she can send distant healing every day. A middle-aged man with his own family may not feel able to offer enough comfort to his younger brother whose twin has committed suicide, but he can send distant healing. A mother whose adult son stopped speaking to her years ago may feel acutely the separation and send distant healing to their relationship and to the grandchildren she has never seen. A corporate manager who senses the sadness of an employee whose wife just suffered a miscarriage may be moved, behind closed doors, to send Reiki to ease his emotional pain.

Hearing the reasons why students have decided to learn Reiki is like looking through a beautiful kaleidoscope at some of the myriad acts of kindness that occur each day in the world. "I'm a social worker, and I want to be able to help the clients I visit during the week. Some of them just aren't doing well." "I have an older dog who has arthritis in his hips, and I want to help him feel better." "My husband just died, so I want to be able to comfort my children, who are pretty upset, and I also want to be able to use Reiki on myself." "My son plays in a junior soccer league, and I'd like to be able to help him recover more quickly whenever he's injured so he can get back in the game." "I'm volunteering at a hospice, and the coordinator recommends that we all learn Reiki. She says that it will help ease our patients' pain and help us deal with stress as well." The list goes on and on, with each individual describing unique challenges and yet echoing the desire to be of service, to offer help, to be kind. It's inspiring simply to listen, as well as instructive: we witness the beauty of the human spirit and realize that our reserves of inner strength and compassion are great.

Yet once we've learned Reiki and begun to practice, it's easy to shrug off the commitment we've made as "no big deal." It's such a little thing to offer Reiki for a few minutes to a coworker who feels a tension headache coming on, or to send Reiki to a shut-in who lives across the street or to a neighbor who fell while shoveling snow and now hobbles around on crutches. It takes so little time and requires only a bit of attention to focus on the client, on the intention to offer healing, and on the flow of the Reiki energy. Yet it is such a powerful act, because it changes the world. In an instant, it is evidence that one human being is willing to set aside distractions to focus on another, to be still in order to stand by another, to be mindful of another's need in order to send healing, to be compassionate without attachment to outcome or expectation of thanks so that another's burdens may be lightened and pain relieved.

Of course, it is the Reiki energy itself that does the healing, that penetrates the diseased tissue, soothes the shattered mind, eases the broken heart, and uplifts the weary spirit again and again, often with such amazing success that physicians and counselors feel challenged to explain the change for the better. Yet the Reiki practitioner's willingness to commit that hour or two to offer a treatment or those few minutes to send Reiki healing should be acknowledged and appreciated. These are noble spiritual acts, however small, however much a part of normal, everyday life they might seem. When we offer Reiki, we offer kindness. When we practice Reiki, we practice kindness.

THE FIRST KINDNESS: USING REIKI TO HEAL YOURSELF

In Toronto, Canada, at the Usui Reiki Ryoho International Conference in fall 2002, I was one of many Reiki masters who had the opportunity to ask Japanese Reiki Master Hiroshi Doi questions about Reiki's early history. Like any student with a serious question, I raised my hand and held it up high. "Did Usui-Sensei first do Reiki on himself when he stubbed his toe on a rock on the way down from the top of Mt. Kurama?" I asked.

Mr. Doi nodded in recognition of the story.

"In the history of Reiki that has been passed along through the Gakkai, is this story also told? Is this the first way that Mikao Usui did Reiki healing? He used it on himself?"

"Yes," Mr. Doi said, nodding again and smiling.[1] First, Mikao Usui used Reiki healing on himself.

Daily Reiki self-treatment supports us in recovering and maintaining our own health, well-being, and happiness, and it prepares us to treat clients effectively. Whether we use Reiki hands-on or distant healing, or a combination of both, self-treatment immerses us in the flow of the energy so that we feel connected to Source, cleansed of negativity and healed of old injuries, and fully present to the moment that opens before us, with all of its opportunities. Beginning the day with some hands-on healing prepares us to meet routine and crisis with clarity and calm; ending the day with our hands resting lightly on our hearts, radiating Reiki energy, heals the smallest hurts and restores us to balance. If we treat ourselves with Reiki each day and take care of our own needs—by getting enough sleep, eating a nutritious diet, enjoying healthy exercise, and engaging in creative expression—the same energy that flows through our hands will be immediately available to us when we treat clients. Daily Reiki self-treatment is a wonderful way to be kind to ourselves, and because it relaxes and restores us, it renews our capacity to offer kindness to others.

The history of Reiki tells us that even if we hope to bring about world healing, we should start by healing ourselves. The author of the Usui Memorial

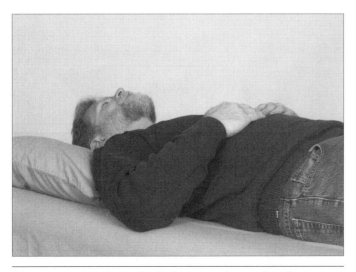

It's easy to get to know the Reiki energy better if we let ourselves relax with hands-on healing at the end of the day.

inscription writes: "To begin spreading the Reiki system, it is important to start from a place close to you (yourself); don't start from something distant, such as philosophy or logic."[2] This emphasis is important. However much we desire to use Reiki to help others, we are to do Reiki on ourselves first; when we want to share Reiki, we will be wise to offer the experience of it rather than attempt to argue or persuade someone to try it. Reiki, which originates in Source, eloquently expresses its own healing nature without need of language or interpretation.

Reiki teachers worldwide continue to reinforce the importance of self-treatment in Reiki I classes, because when the practitioner is well, he or she will be most effective in treating clients. Yet there are other reasons Reiki self-treatment is important: not only does Reiki heal our physical imbalances, but it also gently, gradually heals our emotional, mental, and spiritual wounds, often with such subtlety that we're not even aware of the healing. Only in retrospect do we realize that we are living each day with a more positive attitude, a greater sense of well-being, and an exhilarating awareness of freedom. Reiki self-treatment is one of the cornerstones of practice, and for that reason alone, it should be important to every Reiki practitioner and teacher. Yet it's also one of the easiest ways to give ourselves healing and spiritual growth—and isn't that a kindness?

OBSTACLES TO KINDNESS

When we are committed to Reiki as spiritual practice, not only do we treat ourselves with hands-on or distant healing each day, but we also make an effort to remember and be guided by the Reiki principles. Most of us think often about how to be kind to family members and friends, colleagues and clients, neighbors and acquaintances, and even absolute strangers. We also consider how to be more caring to our pets, farm animals, wildlife, and the earth itself. However, few of us consider the possibility that the fifth principle's encouragement to be kind is meant to be applied to ourselves.

Why? For the last two thousand years, our predominantly Christian culture has placed a high value on martyrdom and self-sacrifice, both noble virtues. If we were raised in a family that accepted and praised these values, we may feel more familiar—and therefore more comfortable—with suffering than with security, prosperity, and abundance. Contemporary culture, rooted more strongly in commercial enterprise than in religion and spirituality, has gone to the opposite extreme. The media offers us celebrities rather than saints and martyrs to emulate, and showcases the lifestyles of the rich, famous, and self-indulgent. Front-page headlines make it clear that few celebrities are happy, despite whatever fame and material wealth they've achieved. Neither attitude—that of self-sacrifice or that of self-indulgence—seems to offer a way to real happiness.

Yet that's the promise of the Reiki principles: "the secret method of inviting happiness." Reiki, which reveals our connection to Spirit and allows us to channel Spirit-guided life-force energy for healing, is compatible with all religions and can enhance our religious experience. However, in helping us appreciate the true essence of religion, Reiki also helps us see what is non-essential and question it. In this gentle way, we gradually become aware that some of the concepts that we've been conditioned to accept through our family and religious heritage are elaborate intellectual constructions, the projections of changing religious philosophies. We can continue to accept them, knowing their flawed nature, or we can shed them, like heavy clothes we no longer need to wear because we feel the warmth of the sun.

One of the ways that Reiki gradually heals us is to restore us to natural balance: physical, mental, emotional, and spiritual. What if the fifth principle, "Just for today, be kind," is intended to encourage us to be kind in balance: not only to others, but also to ourselves? Reiki, with its equal emphasis on self-treatment and client treatment, with its new paradigm of healing, in which both client and practitioner benefit from the flow of energy, gently beckons us forward toward wholeness, well-being, and happiness. Reiki, which draws on an infinite Source for healing, invites us to recognize that there's enough for all of us to experience health, happiness, love, fulfillment, prosperity, and success. There is enough. Because there is enough, it's possible for us to be kind to ourselves without lessening the quality of life for anyone else—and it is wise to learn how to do so.

NOW YOU: KINDNESS IN BALANCE

Becoming more conscious of values that you learned and accepted long ago, as a child raised in a certain family or confirmed in a particular religion, can free you to choose to behave today in a way that reflects your true, authentic nature. In a journal, write down whatever you can remember of family discussions about self-sacrifice. Then turn to memories of religious instruction. What were you taught about self-sacrifice by the clergy? What aspects of this value did you accept and embrace? Sit with these memories and reflections for a while. Are you still living by the same values today? Do you want to do so?

Next, think about self-indulgence. Did your family talk to you about the value of working hard for what you wanted, or were you usually given what you wanted on demand? If your family belonged to a church, synagogue, or mosque, did your religious elders talk to you about the dangers of self-indulgence? Do you regard yourself as being too self-indulgent? Is it possible that you're in the habit of being kind to yourself?

Consider how you begin each day. Write about your routine and what motivates you to follow it. Do you see evidence of too much self-sacrifice? Do you give up eating breakfast each day to make sure that your husband and children have their cereal and scrambled eggs; that their clean clothes, briefcases, and backpacks are in order; and that they get out the door on time? Or do your reflections on your routine make you feel guilty about sleeping through the alarm, drinking too many cups of coffee, being late for work again, or sneaking another cigarette? Over time, self-indulgence is often self-destructive; it's not the same as being kind to yourself.

Think about how to start your day with real kindness, both to yourself and others. What behaviors might you like to change? If you're not already doing Reiki self-treatment, can you wake up a few minutes earlier to give yourself some peace, quiet, and healing to prepare you for the day? Can you take a moment to recite the Reiki principles and remind yourself of the possibility of happiness and healing that they promise? Can you give yourself five minutes just to look out the window and watch the changing colors of dawn? If you awaken and rise with the intention of being mindful of small ways that you might be kind to yourself as well as others, you will discover that the tone of the day changes from strident discord to balanced harmony.

ACCEPTING KINDNESS

Many practitioners are unaccustomed to asking for help and have a difficult time accepting it. Yet there are times when it's essential to accept help and to do so with gratitude and gladness. When we're traumatized, when we've suffered a loss, when life has presented us with a problem with no immediate solutions, we may find that it's for the highest good to simply accept the kindness offered to us.

"Do you remember that snowstorm we had on Tuesday?" my friend Lauren Sage asked, her voice quickening with excitement at what she was about to tell me. I was returning her phone call late on a Saturday afternoon in January, watching out my window as darkness settled over the patches of snow still in the backyard. My left hand cradled the phone against my ear, while my right hand rested lightly over my middle. I felt the gentle flow of Reiki.

"Yes, I remember it," I answered, thinking back to that day, when I watched thick, whirling white flakes through the same window. "I was lucky, though. I didn't have to drive anywhere in it."

"Well, I did," Lauren said, "and coming home from work in that snowstorm, I slid off the road into a ditch. I had no traction. The car ended up pitched at an angle. And it all happened so fast that I stayed calm. I was pretty shaken up the next day though."

"What did you do?"

"I called my husband on my cell phone, but he was at the doctor's office having an outpatient procedure done on his foot. I knew that he wouldn't really be able to help me. Then the most amazing thing happened: as I got off the phone with him, these people came up to my car from all directions—six of them—all offering to help.

"There was a couple from Philadelphia who'd pulled their car over behind mine. There was a man who worked in construction who stopped his truck in front of me and walked back. There was a woman who saw the accident happen through her front window. She bundled up into a coat and went up the street to get her husband and another neighbor to help. They all came to help."

"How wonderful to have so many people show up right at the moment you needed them," I said.

"Yes, I felt really blessed. And they weren't dressed to shovel me out of a ditch or push the back of my car. One woman was in a white coat, and it got all muddy, but she said she didn't care. She just wanted to help. The man who was a construction worker had a set of new chains in his truck, which he put on my tires to give me traction. Between that and everyone pushing, I was back on the road even before my husband drove up. These people were so kind. I felt so protected by the energy."

"I'm sure you were. I've felt the same sense of protection myself."

Then she continued her story: "That night I sent Reiki healing to everyone who had helped me. I was surprised, because the energy was really intense. I think someone in the group really needed healing."

"That was kind of you—and a lovely way to thank them all," I said.

"Well, none of them would take anything. Sending them Reiki seemed a good way to return the kindness."

No matter whether we're beginning practitioners or experienced teachers, we all have times of crises and loss in our lives that can push us to the point of physical and emotional exhaustion. As many practitioners have discovered, such sustained stress depletes us and diminishes our ability to restore ourselves to balance quickly through Reiki. At such times, it's important to acknowledge that we need help and to ask for it. Fortunately, sometimes help comes unasked. Accept all kindness with gratitude. Allow others to experience the joy of giving. Accepting such gifts heals you and reminds you that whatever crisis you've endured, you're at home here on planet Earth—and still among friends.

KINDNESS IN ACTION: INFORMALLY GIVING REIKI TO OTHERS

Practitioners who informally offer Reiki to others, such as a friend in need of headache relief, a child with an upset stomach, or a spouse with severe back pain, channel the same powerful, healing energy as those who are paid for their time. They engage, often quite selflessly, in Reiki as an act of kindness. Is there any way to enhance the quality of such impromptu Reiki sessions?

One simple way is to be sensitive to the client's need for quiet or communication. Someone suffering from a migraine headache may not really want much information about what Reiki is and what it can do to help. It may be enough to say, "Would you like me to do a little hands-on healing?" and nothing more. If the answer is a nod of the head, proceed. However, a friend who has lived with chronic back pain and sought medical treatment from a series of specialists will probably want some explanation of what Reiki is, and may want to see a few hand positions demonstrated before consenting to sit forward on a chair or stool to receive hands-on treatment. If a prospective client is curious but still unsure whether or not to accept the offer of Reiki, ask if you may hold the client's hand to provide a "sample" of some of the sensations he or she might experience during a treatment. This is usually enough to reassure the client of Reiki's safety and gentleness, and it is also likely to make the client eager to experience more.

Once you've both agreed to the treatment, take a moment to assess your client's comfort and that of the setting. If your client is sitting in a chair, is his or her back well supported? If the client lies on a bed or couch, would a pillow under the knees help relieve pressure on the spine? When a bodywork table at

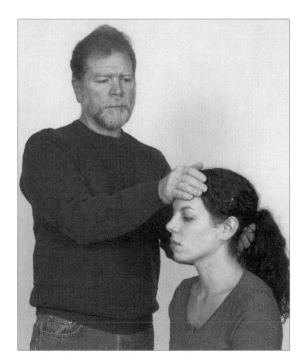

Offering an informal Reiki session is an act of kindness.

the proper height isn't at hand, it's also important to ensure your own comfort, because the energy will first go toward easing any discomfort the practitioner feels before overflowing from the hands. This might mean having a client lie on stacked pillows on the floor rather than the carpet so you don't have to lean, or having the client lie inverted and close to the edge of a bed so you can easily treat the head and front of the torso.

Of course, it isn't always possible to adjust the client's posture or placement. An accident victim thrown clear of a car onto asphalt should not be moved by anyone except paramedics, who can position him or her carefully on a stretcher so that the neck and spine are held motionless en route to the hospital. A Reiki practitioner who is first on the scene may be trained and certified to do first aid, but if not, after calling for help, the practitioner is limited to applying Reiki without moving the client at all. This may mean kneeling on cold, gritty asphalt while holding the client's hand or touching a shoulder. This will not be comfortable for the practitioner, but it is one safe way to deliver Reiki healing to the accident victim within the critical "golden hour," when the body can receive the most benefit from medical help or complementary care. One alternative is for the practitioner to stand back from the accident scene and beam energy or send distant healing—and in some situations (for example, when an accident victim is pinned under wreckage), this is all that is possible. However, if the practitioner makes that choice, the accident victim loses the benefit of the *physical* comfort of touch and the conscious awareness of another human being's kindness.

Even practitioners who live relatively solitary lives sometimes have the opportunity to offer Reiki as kindness to others; for example, a park ranger might offer Reiki to a climber with a broken leg as they wait together for a rescue vehicle to arrive; a beekeeper might use Reiki to quiet a disturbed hive; a reclusive artist, invited into the city for a gallery opening, might discover a companion who would be glad to receive Reiki for headache or heartburn relief. However, for most people who live or work alone, learning distant healing opens up the possibility of using Reiki to bring healing to many more clients. For them, setting aside a half hour to an hour in the morning or evening to do distant healing is a wonderful way to practice Reiki and kindness. The Reiki offered becomes healing meditation and spiritual service.

How can the quality of this experience be enhanced? The practitioner can take care of his or her own comfort. Sitting in a chair that provides good back support helps maintain relaxed awareness and makes it easy to breathe in a meditative way. Placing a glass of springwater close by allows the practitioner to quench thirst if the need arises. Having a notebook and pen available enables the practitioner to record progress notes and jot down any impressions. Quiet solitude encourages focus on the distant-healing session.

It is also a pleasure to do Reiki in a place that feels like a sanctuary. This may be a particular rock under a piñon tree and the desert sky, the back pew of a church or temple, or a comfortable chair in a corner of a bedroom. Natural and man-made sanctuaries are everywhere. And because we can do Reiki anywhere, and with the touch of a hand instantly become more conscious of our connection to Spirit, we can "be in the world but not of it" wherever we are. The bustling airport full of weary travelers, the crowded marketplace, and streets thronged with festival goers can each become a sanctuary when we do Reiki or take a moment to be mindful of the Reiki principles. Yet it is a kindness to ourselves to create within our homes a sacred space of physical beauty and comfort where we can go each day to meditate, pray, and do Reiki. The convenience of this space encourages us to make our spiritual practice part of our daily routine, and our commitment to that practice invites and welcomes Spirit.

LIVING KINDNESS

How can we be kind to others as we go about our lives? If we begin the day with a sense of gratitude for our own lives and for the day itself, this task becomes easier. Why? Gratitude is a feeling of deep appreciation for what is, just as it is. It's an acknowledgment of the good that already exists in our lives. It celebrates the abundance we're experiencing right now. Gratitude warms the heart, and in that warmth, we find that it is easy to be generous with kind thoughts, words, and deeds. When we offer simple kindness, we echo Spirit's kindness to us.

In the sweet mood of gratitude, we find it easy to encourage a child facing a difficult school day; to hold the door open wide for an elderly woman steadying herself with a cane; to put extra coins in the parking meter for the driver who will pull up next; to get coffee for the secretary who usually brings coffee to us; to give our complete attention to the student intern who must master a new task; to send a "thinking of you" card to a friend who's having a difficult time; to walk the dog and take extra time to play fetch in the park; to rub the shoulders of a partner, tired from a long day's work; to volunteer to bake a cake for a church picnic; or to head a committee for a community event.

When we appreciate the blessings in our own lives, we're inclined to think well of others, to put in a good word for someone else, and to do a good deed, even when no one's watching. These actions are natural expressions of a higher consciousness, without self-consciousness. When we deliberately practice gratitude, we become continually more aware and appreciative of Spirit at work in our lives. As a result, we become better able to give and receive kindness.

KINDNESS IN BALANCE: SETTING BOUNDARIES

According to both Western (Usui Shiki Ryoho) and Japanese (Usui Reiki Ryoho) traditional teaching, Mikao Usui practiced kindness. While the story told and retold by Hawayo Takata and the Reiki masters she initiated differs somewhat from the historical account of Usui's life recorded on his memorial at Saihoji Temple in Tokyo, both describe Usui's willingness to offer Reiki to those most in need without thought of reward. Takata's story, however, presented him as having had second thoughts when his selfless service was unappreciated. Usui's encounter with the ungrateful beggar who had returned to his old way of life and to ill health caused him to leave the Beggar City, solicit paying clients, and embrace the Reiki principles.

Many people have interpreted Takata's account as an admonition never to give Reiki away for free, but this seems a simplification of the moral of this tale. Takata described Usui as devoted to his practice of offering Reiki to those in greatest need of healing. He continued to perform this service for years, supported by the Beggar King, until he discovered that his kindness had been unappreciated. Nothing in Takata's account tells us that Usui regretted his years of service or would have taken back a single kind action that he performed, nor does his decision to leave the Beggar City and seek paying clients imply that he would never again offer Reiki for free. Usui was grateful for Reiki's ability to bring healing, and he wanted those who received that healing to be grateful for it as well.

Why, then, did Takata present us with the parable of the ungrateful beggar? Perhaps she wanted to encourage us to practice kindness to others but be kind to ourselves as well. Draining our own resources and reserves in an effort to be kind to others without recognition, reward, or the possibility of replenishment is not healthy but self-destructive. At the very least, it can damage self-respect. If we at least receive simple gratitude in return, we feel acknowledged and supported. In Takata's story, it was when gratitude was absent from the beggar's heart that Usui turned away from him. Takata would have practitioners offering Reiki—or kindness—to unappreciative people set boundaries, say no, and finally turn away. Takata understood that Reiki practitioners must learn to balance kindness to others with a healthy sense of self-worth. In this way, both practitioners and clients can grow into greater wholeness and well-being.

KINDNESS IN ACTION: AT THE REIKI TABLE

Professional practitioners on staff at a holistic center have the privilege of offering several hands-on treatments each day, five or six days a week. The most conscientious offer treatments with mindfulness and appreciation for the healing their clients receive, and that they themselves receive as channels of the Reiki energy. This willingness to be present, sensitive, and caring contributes to the quality of the experience for both clients and practitioners. Fortunately, the flow of the Reiki energy fascinates and focuses the mind and brings a sense of peaceful serenity, making it easy to approach even new clients with kindness.

One simple way to be sensitive to a new client's needs is to schedule time to talk informally, in a relaxed setting outside the treatment room, before the first treatment session begins. After asking the client about his or her general condition, you'll want to make a mental note of the client's answer and then visually assess the client's posture, skin tone, and strength of voice. To help the client feel more comfortable about the prospect of receiving treatment in an unfamiliar modality, you can educate the client by briefly describing Reiki as a gentle form of bodywork and energy medicine that has become well known for bringing a sense of deep relaxation, relieving pain, and accelerating healing. It's worthwhile to reassure the client that during the treatment, he or she will remain fully clothed and will lie down in a comfortable position on a bodywork table in a private room.

You may want to emphasize that during the treatment, the client's comfort and sense of safety are of paramount importance. Lighting, room temperature, background music—or quiet—are the client's choice; blankets can be added for warmth; pillows and bolsters can be used to support the client's head and knees or back; belts, eyeglasses, and shoes can be removed to help ease the client into relaxation. When a practitioner takes the time to describe to a new client "the lay of the land" within the treatment room before they enter together, the client feels empowered to make some choices for his or her own aesthetic pleasure and comfort. This small courtesy also gives the client some sense of control and prepares him or her to simply relax and enjoy receiving the Reiki treatment.

What may help the most to prepare the client is taking a few more minutes, before entering the treatment room, to describe how the Reiki treatment will be done. You may want to demonstrate the pattern of hand positions used in self-treatment and then indicate how the hand positions will be modified for client treatment. You may also want to describe how clients usually perceive the flow of the Reiki energy through a practitioner's hands as warmth, tingling, or a sense of peace and then invite questions. This respects the client's intelligence, and is a beautiful way to acknowledge that you don't take lightly the trust the client places in you as a practitioner and holistic health care provider—and it is also kind.

At this point, it's easy to ask the client to share any health concerns and invite description of any special needs or treatment requests. This establishes a tone of courteous professionalism and caring respect. Some practitioners, particularly those on staff in hospitals or spas, must go a step further and have the client fill out an intake form indicating some of the same information. This may briefly divert the client's attention from the relationship you are developing with one another, but it's essential in many institutional settings for legal and financial reasons. How can you support the client through those few minutes of paperwork? Provide a pen, along with a clipboard for writing, and indicate that you're available for questions. Then allow the client to have a few quiet moments to fill out the necessary forms, while you enter the treatment room, double-check that everything is ready, and invite in the Reiki energy. Beam it around the room through your raised, open hands, or visualize the appropriate Reiki symbols on the walls, floor, and ceiling. Put on the client's choice of music. Adjust the lighting and temperature. Then return to the client, take the form for later filing, and invite the client to enter a place of peace and healing.

At the end of the treatment, ease the client back to ordinary awareness by gently calling his or her name. Once you have a response, you might step out of the room to allow the client some privacy to sit up slowly, get down from the table, slip on shoes, and freshen up. If your client is elderly or needs physical support to get off the table, stay in the room while the client returns

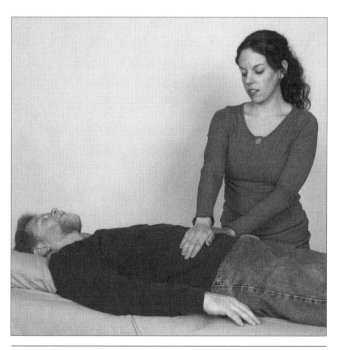

The practitioner's sensitivity to the client's needs is a comforting accompaniment to the relaxing flow of Reiki and offers additional support to the healing process.

191

to a more alert state. Then help the client off the table and stand by, ready to offer a steadying arm or hand. If necessary, provide a footstool for those whose legs don't easily reach the floor, and have a chair close by so the client can sit for a few moments before standing. Some elderly clients will appreciate being handed their eyeglasses and helped into their shoes. If the client is physically disabled, place his or her walker or cane within arm's reach. Honor the uniqueness of the individual before you and, with every gesture, indicate gratitude for the opportunity to treat your client with Reiki.

Returning clients don't need to meet with a practitioner for as long before a treatment, because they are already familiar with the treatment room, the treatment process, and the layout of the facility—and by this time, they are comfortable with the practitioner. However, they will appreciate some time with you to talk about any current concerns and their responses to the previous Reiki session. Particularly, they may want to talk about how long the healing effects lasted and, if they dissipated, why they did so.

When this issue comes up, it's a chance to reinforce the value of repeated treatments in bringing healing to chronic or serious, life-threatening conditions. (My teacher recommended four treatments, in daily succession if possible, to simulate a loading dose of medicine, followed by regularly scheduled treatments convenient for both client and practitioner, perhaps once or twice a week, or every other week.)

This brief conversation before the treatment is also a chance for you and the client to deepen your relationship and for you to answer any of the client's questions about Reiki. Ultimately, you may want to encourage the client to learn Reiki, or the client may ask for information about classes. Being willing and able to provide this information with an encouraging smile, even though it may lessen a client's dependence on you for regular treatments, is kindness—and an indication of the practitioner's trust in Source to provide continued abundance and blessings.

A LAST
CALL FOR KINDNESS

When Barbara Friling smiles, her whole face lights up, and her blue eyes shine with knowing wisdom. She has experienced life as a divorced, single mother and done more than just survive; she has triumphed: she has turned out three adult children who are happy and successful in their own careers, and she has established herself as a sought-after massage therapist, Reiki practitioner, and teacher. She remembers without regret the days, not so long ago, when she worked as a telephone operator at a car dealership and lived in a spare bedroom in her father's house. Those experiences gave her a strong incentive to create a future life that she could love: she chose to learn Reiki, study at the Pennsylvania Institute of Massage Therapy, and move out once a room became available in a friend's house nearer to her work. Finally, certificates and degrees in hand, she made the commitment to rent space at a suburban Philadelphia wellness center contiguous with a long-term care facility, and she bought a townhouse to celebrate her independence and decorated it to reflect the beauty, peace, and joy she now claims every day of her life.

Although Barbara's determination and commitment to do work she loves has transformed her life in many positive ways, her kindness has also brought her many rewards: she is more aware of her own inner strength, has learned the depth of her own compassion, respects and values herself. One of her early experiences with a client proved to be a dramatic turning point in her own life: In fall 2001, a seventy-two-year-old woman, who had been diagnosed with terminal pancreatic cancer and suffered a stroke twenty-four hours later, contacted Barbara to ask for alternative healing care to ease her final days. This woman, a new patient at the long-term care facility, was a recently retired school psychologist with a quick, curious, and open mind. She was fascinated by holistic health care practices and wanted to hire Barbara to do massage, aromatherapy, and Reiki on a daily basis. Barbara soon found that this perceptive, wise woman preferred Reiki over other modalities. Simple, hands-on treatment eased the woman's pain and gave her peace.

After a few weeks of daily Reiki treatments, Barbara's client asked if she could learn to do Reiki on herself, not to replace the treatments Barbara provided but to make the hours in between treatments more comfortable. Barbara taught her bedridden client over two days, giving thorough instruction in self-treatment and repeating the attunements four times to enhance the flow of energy through the woman's hands. Her client delighted in the subtle sensations of warmth and tingling, and discovered that doing hands-on healing enabled her to relax more deeply into rest and sleep between treatments.

Barbara sensed that her client was more comfortable after learning Reiki. Barbara said that over the next week, the woman "seemed better, her appetite was good, and her attitude was positive and peaceful. She smiled a lot and asked even more questions about the work we were doing together." That weekend, some of the client's relatives surprised her with a Halloween visit in costume, which also cheered her up.

Barbara remembers, "Another week and a half went by. By now I was coming to treat her at least once a day, sometimes twice, then I would come back again in the evening just to sit with her after everyone had gone home. I had grown very fond of her. I knew that we'd been together in another lifetime. Perhaps I was now repaying a loving gesture she had made to me in a time long past."

Then a day came when even Barbara's treatments didn't bring her client relief: "I had been to see her three times, and she wasn't feeling well and was getting worse with each visit. The family had been there during the day and evening. I caught up with them around 7:00 p.m., and we all sat with her for a bit. I kissed her goodnight and went home.

"Around 9:00 p.m., I had this desire to go back to see her, so I did. I spoke with the nurses on duty and explained that I wasn't family. They said they knew but that it was okay for me to be there. So I went into her room, sat beside her, and for the next four and a half hours, used Reiki. I had often wondered why I had taken the Reiki classes. During those hours with her, I knew why—and I was so very grateful. I did hands-on Reiki, sent distant healing, and worked in her aura. Occasionally she would stir, notice that I was there, and then drift away again. Her breathing was labored, and the room was heavy with angels hovering nearby. It was amazingly peaceful.

"Holding her hand and doing Reiki, I continued to remind her that everything was okay, that she was loved beyond measure, that she wasn't alone, that I loved her dearly, and that it was okay to go to friends or family if she saw them or into the light if she felt drawn to it. In her final moments, she became very calm and peaceful. She took her last breath, and I stayed with her, just holding her in my arms, for another half hour."

As Barbara walked out of the building into the parking lot, she looked up at the beautiful full moon lighting the night sky and felt a happy child-like presence with her. "This is incredible," she heard her client's voice say. "Thank you." Barbara found herself speechless, smiling and crying as her heart overflowed with joy and gratitude that she had been privileged to witness the gentle transition of this soul.

NOW YOU: STAND BY ME

Some Reiki practitioners choose professions or volunteer activities that allow them to sit at the bedside of the dying. Reiki-trained geriatric and critical-care nurses, social workers, and hospice volunteers have the opportunity to practice Reiki on patients whose days and hours are numbered. Such patients are often enormously grateful for the care, consideration, and kindness of those who tend to their needs. Whether or not the patients can express this gratitude in words, the practitioners have the satisfaction of knowing that they've comforted the sick, eased someone's pain, and offered a sense of peace to the dying.

Most Reiki practitioners aren't faced with death on a daily basis. Yet we may be asked by a client to be present in that final hour of need, we may choose to be at the bedside of a dying friend or relative, or we may find that we're the only one nearby when someone draws that last breath. What should we do? The answer is simple: stay, give comfort, and offer Reiki.

If you have never faced this task, you may worry that you won't be able to marshal your inner strength and courage to do what is right. So many of us fear dying; so many more fear the ugliness and indignity of the suffering that precedes death. We suffer with the dying. How can we bear to be with the dying in that last moment as they leave the physical world and enter the invisible realm of Spirit? We make a choice to put all our own fears and worries aside, to be fully present, and to be kind.

Each day, in every encounter, we have the same choice, although the consequences don't seem so momentous when we're less aware of time running out. Each day, we can choose to put aside our concerns and be kind to the cloakroom attendant we've never seen before and won't see again, to the waitress who is new on the job and nervous, and to the taxicab driver who knows so little English that we wonder if he can read a street map. Sooner or later, death is coming to us all. Let that knowledge compel us to be more compassionate, to be kind.

MIKAO USUI: KINDNESS AS A WAY OF BEING

The Usui Memorial, outside Saihoji Temple in Tokyo, is a very tall stone inscribed with many columns of Japanese calligraphy that offer a fairly complete account of Mikao Usui's life written by one of his students soon after his death in March 1926. About midway through the inscription, which was first translated and published in English in Frank Arjava Petter's *Reiki Fire: New Information about the Origins of the Reiki Power; A Complete Manual,* the author describes Usui's experience on Mt. Kurama.

> One day he went to Mount Kurama on a 21-day retreat to fast and meditate. At the end of this period he suddenly felt the great Reiki energy at the top of his head, which led to the Reiki healing system. He first used Reiki on himself, then tried it on his family. Since it worked well for various ailments, he decided to share this knowledge with the public at large. He opened a clinic in Harajuku, Aoyama—Tokyo—in April of the 11th year of the Taisho period (*in 1921*). He not only gave treatment to countless patients . . . but he hosted workshops to spread his knowledge. In September of the twelfth year of the Taisho period (*1923*), the devastating Kanto earthquake shook Tokyo. Thousands were killed, injured, or became sick in its aftermath. Dr. Usui grieved for his people, but he also took Reiki to the devastated city and used its healing powers on the surviving victims.[2]

This account records how Mikao Usui used Reiki: first on himself, then to treat willing family members, and then to offer healing to "the public at large." Although he might have chosen to keep Reiki a precious secret, a family treasure to be passed on like a jewel from generation to generation, instead he chose to share Reiki's many blessings.

Usui established clinics where he certainly had paying patients, but the author of the account particularly praises his volunteer work, searching through the earthquake rubble to give Reiki freely to the sick, injured, and dying. The selflessness with which he ministered to those affected by the Kanto earthquake in the days and weeks that followed the devastation is evidence of a deeply compassionate mind and heart.

This account describes Mikao Usui as someone who practiced kindness as a way of being. In addition to his work as a healer and spiritual teacher, he took time each morning and night to meditate on the Reiki principles, and he recommended that others do the same. He valued the power of human kindness so much that he focused his complete attention on it at the beginning and end of each day. For someone so committed to bringing healing to his own life and to the world, perhaps this was the most natural choice. As practitioners of Reiki, we can learn to make the same choice. As Mikao Usui asked, we can focus on the inner light of kindness, and in doing so, kindle its flame so that it burns brightly within us, guiding our actions and lighting our way.

KINDNESS IN ACTION: VOLUNTEERING

Many Reiki practitioners discover that their enjoyment of practice awakens in them the desire to offer Reiki more often and to more people. After doing Reiki on themselves and a few family members and friends for months or years, they decide that they really want to do more, so they look for volunteer opportunities. Although in some states, license-to-touch laws can restrict opportunities for hands-on healing to those who meet certain credentialing requirements, certified practitioners can still offer Reiki using the same hand positions used during a formal client treatment, elevated a few inches *above* the body, in the energy field. This complies with the law and is highly effective as a way to channel Reiki healing energy. In states without such laws, Reiki practitioner-volunteers are actively sought, particularly to work in hospices. Other venues that often welcome Reiki practitioner-volunteers include hospitals, long-term care facilities, wellness centers, community-run counseling centers, and charity-benefit sporting events.

Another way that Reiki practitioners may satisfy their appetite for volunteering and gain wider experience in client treatment is to participate in an ongoing Reikishare or healing circle; and if one doesn't exist locally, they may establish one. This isn't as difficult to do as it might sound: it requires an adequate space, one or more bodywork tables, and one or more practitioners willing to offer Reiki to others for an hour or two at no charge, or for a small donation (to pay for the space, if necessary). Fortunately, Reiki practitioners in a single class may discover that a classmate is willing to donate the use of a basement or spare room on a regular basis. For example, a practitioner might volunteer to host a Reikishare every other Wednesday night or the second Sunday afternoon each month. At that time, practitioners arrange to meet for a couple of hours to practice Reiki on one another. To ensure that everyone receives Reiki, practitioners may agree to limit treatment time to twenty minutes per person or limit treatment to standard positions on the front or back of the body.

Reiki masters who teach frequently sometimes coordinate Reikishares at locations where they hold classes. This is an excellent way to support new practitioners in developing a more refined perception of the subtle sensations of the Reiki energy, and it also fosters a sense of community among more experienced practitioners. Some Reiki masters welcome members of the general public. When this is the case, it's important to have someone available to stay with the newcomers, ready to provide a brief introduction to Reiki and answer any questions that arise.

After about a dozen years participating in and coordinating Reikishares, I've found that I like to begin the share with a welcoming circle to allow those attending to introduce themselves by first name and briefly describe how they feel. After introductions and any community announcements, we join hands, sending the energy around the circle. Then we go to the bodywork tables, where three to five practitioners work on one client at the same time. During treatment time, we remain silent to allow the client the deepest relaxation and rest. However, directly before and after treatment, there is often a bit of conversation: the mention of special treatment needs; the expression of thanks; description of an intuitive impression. By the end of the three-hour gathering, everyone seems to feel better, happier, and more relaxed—and the sense of community that we've come to share is even stronger.

Before starting a Reikishare, do some soul searching: it's important to be honest with yourself about how much time you have available, how much personal energy you're willing to commit, and how you can best support your local community of Reiki practitioners, both in the short and long term. Be an enthusiastic volunteer, but also be realistic. Don't take on more than you can do, and be willing to ask for help. Sharing the responsibility of hosting or coordinating a Reikishare lightens your workload and invites in more Reiki energy. The commitment to a sustainable community support effort is a kindness to all.

If you decide that you're not able to devote the quantity of time and energy necessary to start and maintain a Reikishare, or to be a regular member, consider offering just one person a complete Reiki treatment as an act of kindness. This might be an elderly neighbor with health problems, a young mother who never takes time for herself, or a troubled teenager who needs some TLC to get through a difficult time. When you see how much your kindness is appreciated, you may decide to continue offering treatments on a regular basis to help this individual through a crisis—and then encourage him or her to learn Reiki. You might also volunteer to treat another Reiki practitioner or teacher who seems particularly tired or stressed out by life's challenges; it's a joy to offer such a treatment, and it is bliss to receive such a kindness, for both giving and receiving Reiki bring healing that rebalances the body, renews energy, and invites gratitude.

ONE VOLUNTEER'S STORY:
THE UNBROKEN CIRCLE
OF KINDNESS

In 1998, a day before her fifty-fifth birthday, Noreen Ryen was diagnosed with bladder cancer. Noreen had been widowed five years before when her husband had undergone the same surgery she now faced. Now she prayed for courage and inner strength to face the ordeal. She agreed to have the operation, but after the surgery, follow-up tests revealed that some cancer remained. So she continued to pray, not only for courage but also for acceptance. Over the next four years, she underwent an additional seven transurethral resections, nine cystoscopies, and three separate rounds of chemotherapy. She also explored alternative and complementary therapies, including meditation and guided visualization, supplemented her diet with vitamins, and learned Reiki. "I used Reiki on myself whenever I had a few minutes," she says. "I fell asleep with my hands covering my lower abdominal area."

During this time, despite her illness and the difficult course of treatment, Noreen continued to work full-time as a certified massage therapist and to volunteer at two locations: a thrift shop that benefits battered women and a wellness center for cancer survivors. "People have always been so kind to me," she says. "I just wanted to give something back."

In May 2001, her surgeon advised her to have her bladder removed to prevent possible spread of the cancer to other organs. After many hours of reflection and more prayer, she agreed to the operation. During the surgery, there were complications and a significant loss of blood. Afterward, she spent long weeks in the hospital, feeling as if her life was ebbing away. Then two Reiki friends made a visit. Noreen appreciated their kindness. "I know in my heart that their Reiki treatment that day saved my life and set the pace for my recovery," she says. "I surrendered myself that day and felt the power of that treatment."

Once discharged from the hospital, she was under doctor's orders not to return to work until she had fully recovered her strength. So instead, she spent more time in the thrift store as a volunteer, tending the cash register. "One Saturday afternoon, a gentleman purchased some used furniture for a family who were down on their luck," she recalls. "He gave me a blank check in payment and told me to have the director fill in the amount. I objected, because I didn't want to take the responsibility. I didn't know how many hands the check would go through, and thought it unsafe. The man laughed and said that there was plenty of money in the account. He told me that he wasn't worried that the check wouldn't reach the director's hand. He said he trusted me and left the store." The man's kindness, generosity, and pleasant manner made an impression on Noreen, and her twinkling blue eyes and warm smile stayed with him.

Six months later, the director feigned acceptance of a benefactor's invitation to coffee at closing time, then begged off at the last minute to give the gentleman who'd entrusted the check to Noreen an opportunity to meet her and talk with her. "Noreen will go with you," the director told him, when he walked through the door. "Won't you, Noreen?" The director's matchmaking efforts paid off. In the coffee shop, Bryan and Noreen discovered that they had a lot in common. He invited her for a walk in the park the following weekend, and she says, "The rest is history."

Well, not quite. Bryan knew almost immediately that he wanted to spend the rest of his life with Noreen, but she wasn't so sure. Noreen recalls, "Before consenting to the last surgery, I had resigned myself to living my life alone, and I was really okay with that. I had family and friends, and I was content. I had a comfortable home, a job, and my volunteer work. I didn't know what to make of this new development, and I was unsure how to speak of my health history and the new body image I was learning to accept."

Over the next several months, Bryan courted Noreen. Meanwhile, she went back to work and also pursued her Reiki master training. One weekend, much to the delight of her fellow Reiki practitioners and teacher, she hosted the Reiki master class in her home. There were vases of red roses everywhere. Bryan had sent her a dozen a day. As her classmates admired the bouquets, she protested, "It looks like a funeral parlor in here!" She was embarrassed at having a beau. When asked about her suitor, she simply shook her head, still unsure what to do.

Finally, she decided to talk to Bryan about her health history. "I needn't have worried," she says. "Bryan was just fine with it. He confided that the director had told him a little about my past even before that first cup of coffee. He wanted to meet me and have the chance to get to know me anyway. Imagine that! A man who could be comfortable with me in my post-surgery state, when I doubted anyone could."

Two months later, the weekend of her birthday, Noreen hosted another meeting of the Reiki master class. This time, Bryan dropped in to say hello to us all—wearing a bright yellow tuxedo, a two-foot-high yellow top hat, and a cheery smile. Everyone laughed at his costume and enjoyed the obvious compliment to Noreen. He would be by later, he promised her, to take her out for a celebration with her family.

Six years later, Noreen and Bryan are together, spending much of their time traveling around the United States in an RV with their cat, Earl Gray. "Our families know and like each other, and manage an annual get-together," Noreen says. "We thank God for the gift of each day and for all the wonderful people who have offered Reiki over the years." Noreen, who completed her training as a Reiki master, also finds that she can sometimes find opportunities to offer Reiki to friends met on the road.

And how do she and Bryan best like to spend their days together? Volunteering! Each year, they stay for months at a time at construction job sites in Alabama and Louisiana, working on crews for Habitat for Humanity. They measure and cut wood, swing hammers, and paint drywall and trim to help build houses for Hurricane Katrina survivors, so they can rebuild their lives. And sometimes, at the end of the day, Noreen does a little massage and Reiki on the shoulders of her fellow volunteers.

NOW YOU: DISCOVER WAYS TO GIVE

Although giving Reiki to someone in need is a wonderful way to bring healing and comfort, Reiki enhances the quality of life even beyond the bodywork table. When we volunteer to cook at a community picnic, to make signs advertising a fund-raising event for a good cause, to knit socks for enlisted personnel, or to tutor at a literacy center, our efforts are made more healing by Reiki energy. When we are kind, we're practicing Reiki, so why should we be surprised when our hands become suffused with warmth as we flip pancakes, touch a keyboard, or sign a check to donate to a good cause? Reiki helps us to become more aware of our connection to Spirit and to one another through the energy—and through the practice of kindness.

Discover for yourself a volunteer activity that suits your personality, skills, and schedule and then enjoy giving what you can. Don't look for any reward beyond the satisfaction of knowing that, just as others have been kind to you, you are now able to be kind. The message of kindness—and what it tells about the human heart—is meant to be passed along.

KINDNESS TO THE EARTH

Nature nurtures and renews us, day after day, season after season, because universal life-force energy flows through all of nature. Our impact on the cycles of nature, especially since the industrial age, has put the lives of many creatures in peril. Our own lives, although not immediately threatened, are affected, and the survival of many species, including our own, is at risk.

One way to begin to rectify the imbalances that we've created—and to be kind—is to send distant healing to the earth. A simple method you can do even if you're a newly trained Reiki I practitioner is to raise your Reiki-charged hands to heart level, as if to pray, and then spread them a few inches apart with palms facing each other, imagining the earth, small enough to hold, floating in the space between your palms. Then just listen to your hands, lowering them when the flow of energy finally stops. If you would like, say a prayer for Earth's healing as you send Reiki, or if you're not comfortable saying a prayer, open your heart and send your love, along with the Reiki energy. Listen to the flow, and lower your hands when it ceases.

If you're a trained Reiki II practitioner or a Reiki master, you've learned symbols and methods that enable you to send distant healing to the earth in a more formal and focused way. You can "target" a particular geographic area, such as the Amazon rainforest or the North Atlantic. You can direct energy to support a specific endangered species or ecosystem. You can send Reiki back

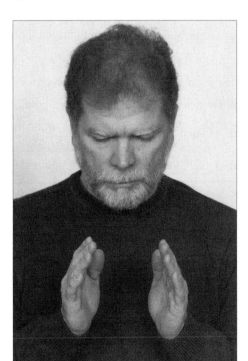

Sending distant healing to the earth

in time to mitigate the environmental damage of toxic waste dumped into the oceans or forward in time to help provide extended protection from global warming. Yes, you can.

Though it's an enormous job and your contribution can only be a small one, with millions of Reiki practitioners sending Reiki even for just a few minutes to the earth every day, there will be healing. Do you remember your first miracle? Do you remember how astonished you were at the degree of healing that occurred? Allow the possibility of healing the whole earth—as predicted in the Usui Memorial—and take a few minutes each day to send Reiki. Whatever other efforts you make to be mindful of our planet's resources, make this effort to be kind to renew life-force energy and restore the earth to natural balance.

A MEDITATION ON KINDNESS

Kindness is an abiding, caring presence. She sits at your bedside when you are ill, holding your hand as you sleep. Kindness holds a cool washcloth against your hot forehead, comforts you as you wake from disorienting dreams, and offers cup after cup of water to help bring your fever down.

Or Kindness sits at your bedside and reads aloud until you relax into sleep. Then he turns out the lamp and withdraws to sleep close by, under a blanket in a chair, within hearing range of a whispered call for help. Or Kindness may sleep in the same bed, ready to awaken you from a nightmare and reassure you that you were only having a bad dream.

Kindness may tell you over lunch, "I don't care what time of day or night it is. Call me, and I will come. I mean it. I will be there for you." Kindness is always willing to be there in the middle of the night for car trouble, early babies, muggings, abandonment, accidents, abuse, pain, fear, and loneliness.

Kindness keeps you company, celebrating your birthday and all the holidays with you when you have just lost a partner, parent, child, or pet. Kindness gently offers you her complex attention. She is willing to listen to whatever you have to say, to hear whatever you need to express—even when you are speechless with grief or fury and all you can utter is a wild howl or moan.

Kindness anticipates your needs. He wraps a blanket around you, even before you realize that you're cold. Kindness puts an arm around your shoulders, leads you to safety, and then turns you so that your back is to the blazing fire burning down your home.

Kindness brings you hot coffee in a thermos cup, sweetened with milk and sugar, and then smiles with concern: "Do you need a doctor? Do you have a place to stay tonight? Let me help you."

It is Kindness that searches the rubble for survivors—and for the dead so that they may be remembered and their lives celebrated by those they've left behind. It is Kindness that turns over the crumbled bricks and stones, and pushes away the fallen timbers in search of the source of that whimper—and Kindness that rejoices to find a family pet or free a frightened child.

It is Kindness that volunteers to help rebuild the house, neighborhood, town, roads, and waterways. It is Kindness that turns the disaster into a journey of discovery for those recovering, an opportunity to explore and understand the compassionate nature of the human heart.

Kindness is capable of offering caring presence even from far away. Kindness sends care packages, calls long distance to other countries, and e-mails often with words of encouragement. And when nothing but physical presence will do, Kindness catches the red-eye or drives the distance.

Kindness may be offered to you by a friend, a family member, a coworker, a colleague, a chat-room acquaintance, or someone you have never met. Kindness knows how to stand by without standing out or standing too far away. Kindness understands the innate dignity of every human being and doesn't overwhelm or embarrass that dignity with excessiveness.

Kindness recognizes and appreciates you just as you are, even when you don't appreciate yourself much. Kindness admires every human being's ability to grow through challenges and struggles, and encourages you to look within to find your strength. Kindness appreciates honest self-assessment, approves your good choices, and rejoices in your accomplishments.

Kindness doesn't judge or condemn you for poor choices made in the past but stands rooted in the present moment, the moment of power and possibility, as steady as the steel pylons that anchor a bridge over turbulent water. "I am here with you *now!*" Kindness says. "You can walk across the bridge from past to future *now*. Let the past go. Make new, better choices. Look forward. I will walk with you."

SUMMARY

For most Reiki practitioners, kindness and compassion come very naturally. If not, experience with the Reiki energy quickly teaches these virtues. Reiki flows through our hands, delivering the precise dose of universal life-force energy necessary to accelerate the client's healing. As practitioners, we witness the powerful effects of this intelligent, dynamic, healing flow and come to appreciate the opportunity to stand by the client—to be a caring, abiding presence, sensitive to another's needs—for the duration of the treatment.

The fifth Reiki principle also encourages us to find ways to practice kindness in our lives: as we do self-treatment; as we treat clients, formally and informally; and as we go about each day, encountering friends, meeting acquaintances, and interacting with strangers. We can practice kindness as a revolutionary act, knowing that it will warm the heart of another soul, who will then pass along the light of kindness.

MORE SUGGESTIONS FOR PRACTICE

❧ After twenty-one years of practice and fourteen years of teaching, I am acutely aware that even the most well-intentioned and professional Reiki practitioners are prone to neglect their own health, well-being, and happiness, putting others' needs first. This is contrary to the way Mikao Usui practiced Reiki, the recommendations inscribed on his memorial stone in Japan, and Takata's practice and recommendations. Without doing Reiki self-treatment or providing adequate self-care, Reiki practitioners can burn out! While this isn't a permanent condition, isn't it better to avoid it altogether?

Take a few moments to consider your own practice: do you begin or end each day by treating yourself with some hands-on healing? If you're a Reiki II practitioner, are you in the habit of sending Reiki to yourself? Do you allow yourself to send Reiki into the past to help you release and forgive situations that caused you pain? When you have a dentist's or doctor's appointment scheduled, do you send Reiki ahead to help the visit go well? Can you commit more time to treating yourself, with hands-on or distant healing, as an act of kindness?

❧ If you feel uncomfortable with the recommendation to make your own healing a higher priority, ask yourself why. If your answer is that you feel guilty or selfish taking time to treat yourself when others need treatment, perhaps you need to consider the nature of the Reiki energy. Are you afraid that there isn't enough to go around? Is that idea based on your experiences with the Reiki energy, or does it derive from some other source? If the idea of lack stems from childhood or cultural conditioning, you may want to discard it. If you recognize that your thoughts of lack are arising from that conditioning, stop them! Substitute thoughts that affirm the abundance of healing energy available to you and everyone through Spirit or Source. Repeat this practice as often as necessary to change your mind and shift your awareness.

Another reason you might feel uncomfortable making your own healing a priority is low self-esteem, an emotional and mental issue that requires healing. If you recognize this as the source of your resistance, be kind to yourself: do Reiki on yourself each day, using either hands-on or distant healing, and let the energy dissolve any habitual feelings of low self-worth. This will uplift you and help you feel more comfortable inviting and accepting happiness.

❧ Think about your daily routine. Is there something you might add or subtract from it in an effort to be kinder to yourself? Would waking up fifteen minutes earlier to fix yourself a healthy breakfast improve your sense of physical well-being, your energy levels throughout the morning, and your mood? Would ten minutes of yoga after work help you relax from your commute? Would committing to call a faraway loved one more often make you both feel happier with your lives? Even if you make only small changes, slowly incorporating them into your life, you will find that you are more content. Life itself will seem kinder to you when you make the effort to be kind to yourself.

❧ In informal situations, offer Reiki generously to others out of kindness, but don't push it on anyone. Let the experience speak for itself. Your clients will thank you for the relaxation and relief from pain that they feel—and, often, they'll want to know more about Reiki. If not, that's okay. It's kind to recognize and honor the uniqueness of each person's life journey.

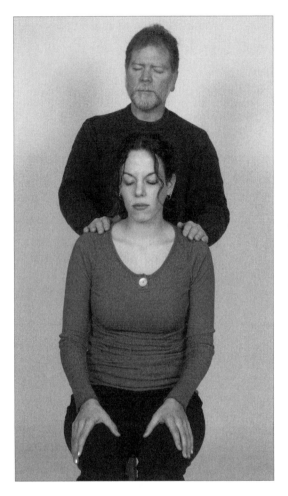

Offer Reiki generously to others in informal situations.

❧ Start practicing "random acts of kindness." Look for ways to surprise friends, family members, acquaintances, and absolute strangers with beauty, laughter, and a sense of abundance. Bring flowers to someone who doesn't expect them. Drop off gently used magazines and books for a hospital patient. Volunteer to paint props for the local theater. Serve Thanksgiving dinner to the homeless in a soup kitchen. Cover the cost of a cup of coffee for the person behind you in line. Return the wallet or purse that was left by accident under the chair. Offer your arm to support the octogenarian called upon to rise and make a toast. Help the child struggling to get into a coat or put on rain boots. Reach out to others to help in small ways, respecting their need for independence, recognizing all you have in common, and sharing the warmth of a smile.

8

THE DOUBLE TITLE

An Invitation to Happiness and a Promise of Miracles

Writing in Japanese calligraphy, Mikao Usui gave two titles to the Reiki principles: "The Secret Method of Inviting Happiness/The Miracle Medicine for All Diseases." What a bold promise he makes to those who practice Reiki! What a marvelous puzzle he leaves us to work out! By presenting the five principles (apparently adopted from Dr. Bizan's book, "A Path to Soundness") with this double title, Usui encourages us to meditate on the principles and do energy healing so that we may come to know both happiness and health.[1]

The two titles are inextricably bound together. Reiki practitioners and teachers around the world are familiar with miracles, which occur with surprising frequency when we do Reiki energy healing, but are we as well acquainted with happiness? We're happy to be able to bring healing to others, and we're happy when we ourselves receive healing. Is there more to "inviting happiness" than doing Reiki hands-on and distant healing? Yes. Mikao Usui concluded this message to his followers with a recommendation to recite the principles twice each day, morning and night, before signing his name and title, "The Founder."

In Japan, traditionally taught Reiki practitioners and teachers (initiated within the Usui Reiki Ryoho Gakkai, the Reiki learning society in existence since Usui's time), generally follow this recommendation. They see Reiki as a spiritual discipline as well as a healing practice. Recognizing it as a way to enlightenment, they chant the principles each day, and also practice meditations that help them focus on the energy. In the West, however, practitioners and teachers have generally been taught to focus on Reiki healing techniques and to see the principles as a set of concepts that Mikao Usui adopted for meditation because of the healthy values they express. As a result, most practitioners here have aimed simply to remember the principles. Yet many of us have come to appreciate them, having learned that being mindful of the principles throughout the day works well to help us navigate through difficult times.

THE REWARDS OF
SURRENDERING THE OUTCOME

In fall 2006, Lauren Bissett brought a friend to a Reikishare at the Dreamcatcher in Skippack, Pennsylvania. She was excited. She had never before invited someone to accompany her. Her family had been supportive of her involvement in Reiki, and her boyfriend tolerant, but no one close to her had said, "Yes, I would like to learn more." The previous day, Lauren had met Alexis McVeigh, a friend from elementary-school days, whom she hadn't seen in years. At the Reikishare, Alexis sat beside Lauren during the opening circle. After she introduced herself, Alexis said she had known about Reiki for years and had even had one Reiki treatment but never felt it was the right time to take a class. Maybe now that she had run into Lauren, she would. Alexis seemed to enjoy the Reikishare, both her time on the table and the chance to participate in hands-on healing. As she went out the door, she waved and said, "See you soon."

Months went by, and Lauren became immersed in her nursing courses and was busy on weekends with Reiki master training and assisting at classes. In addition, she worked part time as a waitress at a diner to pay her rent and school bills. I asked her if Alexis had been in touch. She shrugged and responded, "I haven't seen her. I thought she would follow up on her own about taking a class, but I guess it still isn't the right time."

I felt disappointed for her sake. I thought it would have meant a lot to her to have an old friend join her in practicing Reiki. When my two best friends expressed interest and took classes soon after me, I felt as if I were being joined on an adventure to an exotic land. It was great to be able to explore together and share some experiences with Reiki.

Then in fall 2007, Alexis returned to the Reikishare by herself. She had decided that she wanted to take Reiki I and asked about upcoming classes. Meanwhile, Lauren was busy with her nursing studies during the week and working weekends. It didn't occur to me to let her know that Alexis planned to take a Reiki class.

When Lauren called, it was to talk about her brother, who'd been having personal problems. She had done her best to provide emotional support and had done Reiki to help him with depression. She felt pleased that she had been able to set appropriate boundaries with him, recognizing that he had to want emotional healing for himself. She was also proud that she'd maintained her grades and gone to all her classes, despite the difficulties at home. We talked two or three times by phone. She asked me to put her brother's name on the distant-healing request list that I send out to students and Reiki friends. She had secured his permission.

"How would you like your own name placed on the list? Couldn't you use a bit of support?"

Lauren laughed. "Oh, yeah, that would be good," she said. "You can put my name on the list. It's almost time for finals, and I always do really well when people have sent me Reiki!"

"Okay, you're on!" I teased.

In December 2007, she called me again. "My brother wants to learn Reiki. He says that he wants to be able to use it on himself! I'm so happy," she said. "I know this will really help him."

"That's wonderful! Will you come to the class to assist?"

"Yes. I think he'll feel a little more comfortable with me there. Besides, I would really like to be in the energy of the class. I could use a boost after exam week."

"I'll look forward to seeing you both then."

The following Saturday morning, the students came in out of the cold, one by one. Alexis McVeigh was tucking away her coat and bag when Lauren arrived without her brother. She looked tired and sad. She took me aside and asked, "Did you get my message?"

I nodded. "I'm so sorry he decided not to come."

"Well, it's his choice. I wanted to be here, so I'm here. I'll enjoy being in the energy of the class." She glanced around at the other students, and her mouth opened in a little *o* of surprise. "That's Alexis. That's my friend, Alexis!" She broke into a wide smile.

Alexis turned at the mention of her name and smiled back.

When we commit to Reiki practice and make hands-on healing on ourselves and distant healing on others part of our daily routine, we're in and out of the energy like swimmers running under a waterfall to dive into a pool warmed by sunlight. We're cleansed, day after day, of any negativity that we might have absorbed from people around us or places we have visited, and we're washed clean of our own negative feelings of anger and worry soon after they arise. Remembering the Reiki principles speeds this process.

As we give less personal energy and attention to anger and worry, we need less healing. When we let go of disappointment, frustration, or concern, go on with our lives, and do the best we can, the energy can work on other levels. When we let go of our attachment to a particular outcome, the energy can heal the situation we've surrendered as beyond our conscious control in ways that we never imagined possible.

The first two Reiki principles advise us, "Just for today, do not anger . . . do not worry." These are gentle recommendations. They hint that when we surrender the outcome of a difficult situation to Spirit or Source, events may unfold in more positive ways than we thought possible. We're invited to trust the energy more deeply, to extend the trust we learn through hands-on and distant healing to the Source of that healing throughout the day. We're encouraged to become more conscious and aware of our constant connection to Source. When that awareness becomes integrated into our worldview, we live our lives with a sense of trust in the universe that is beyond faith. We feel comforted by the presence of Spirit. We feel loved, guided, and protected—and content with our lives, just as they are.

A HAPPY MAN

Bob Rowlands says that Reiki has transformed his life. His daughter, Jessica, whose diagnosis of leukemia motivated him to take his first class, has now been in remission for three years. The rest of his family is well, and he considers himself a happy man. He does daily hands-on and distant healing, is mindful of the Reiki principles, and uses affirmations to reinforce his own happiness and that of his wife, son, and daughter. The Reiki principle that he calls to mind most often is gratitude.

At least three times a day, he reflects on the many blessings of his life, giving thanks for all the good in his life now and all the good that's on its way to him. Although he may not know the particulars—who he'll meet or what will happen to bring him an opportunity or touch him with kindness—he expresses his appreciation for these people and events as well. He also envisions the future that he would like to create for himself and his family in as much detail as he can, and then allows his heart to fill with gratitude. Then he lets the vision go, with thanks to Spirit for manifesting this future or an even better one.

He says that he is happily surprised again and again by the unfolding of events in his life. He enjoys using the principle of gratitude and the metaphysical law of "like attracts like" to ensure increased prosperity and success at work, and continued good health, well-being, and happiness at home. Someday, he hopes to have his own holistic center where he can do Reiki treatments and teach classes full-time. He expects to employ the same spiritual tools to build his dream from the ground up and make his holistic center a place of healing and peace, and a business success.

Many Reiki practitioners and teachers were happy with the message of Rhonda Byrne's bestselling book, *The Secret*. Reiki teaches us so much about how the mind influences the body; we can readily understand that our thoughts help create our experience of the world. We can interpret the first Reiki principle, "Just for today, do not anger," as an invitation to stop the negative thoughts and feelings of anger, and replace them with positive thoughts and feelings. We can interpret the second Reiki principle, "Just for today, do not worry," in the same way. If we practice this technique of stopping negative thoughts and replacing them with positive thoughts, we alter our perception *and* our reality. This is good spiritual work.

When we refuse to be drawn into the whirlpool of negativity and instead remain in our peaceful center, aware of the Reiki energy and conscious of our connection to Spirit, we discover that it's easy to feel grateful. Life itself is a profound blessing, and we who have learned Reiki have the most amazing lives! We witness miracles, large and small. The gratitude we feel for Reiki and for our lives magnetizes more of that for which we feel grateful—loving relationships, good work, healing, health, well-being, prosperity, success, fulfillment, and happiness.

FALLING IN LOVE WITH LIFE

Karen Thompson and I lingered to talk after a Reikishare at the Dreamcatcher. She had assisted at the Reiki I class there the previous day, for no other reason than that she just loved "being in the energy." She told me she'd had an impression during the attunements that she wanted to share. "Do you remember talking about how, after you learned Reiki, you wished you could have more hands?" she asked.

I laughed and nodded. I did remember.

"Well, during one of the attunements, I had this impression as I was beaming energy to the circle. I saw everyone's hands coming together in the center of the circle to do healing, one by one, as you attuned each person. Then there were more and more hands. There were infinite hands coming together to do healing. I think you've gotten your wish." She grinned.

"Thank you," I told her, because the impression she had just shared validated so many of my hopes as a teacher.

"Thank you! You have no idea how excited I was just to be there. It felt so good to be in the energy and to be with so many people who were experiencing the energy for the first time. I felt so happy—and it's carried over to today. I've been feeling happy more and more of the time."

I was quiet, enjoying her enthusiasm. It was my turn to encourage her with her work: psychotherapy, hypnotherapy, and Reiki. We talked for a few minutes about places where she might do introductory talks or demonstrations—libraries, hospitals, or local chambers of commerce. She was excited about all the opportunities that were unfolding in her life.

Then, for a moment, she looked almost wistful. "Do you remember a few years ago, when I first started Reiki? Do you remember how indifferent I was to life?"

I remembered and was surprised, not by the recollection but by the contrast between this dynamic, enthusiastic woman and my memory of her as a beginning Reiki student: beautiful and gifted but sad and apathetic. "Yes," I said, nodding.

"I didn't really want to be here then, alive on this planet."

"I know."

"Now I'm glad to be here. I accept being here. I embrace it. I love my life! Who could have imagined how much my life would change, how much I would change, because of Reiki?"

There was nothing I could say in response. She knew that the changes in her life were the result of her own spiritual growth. This was something she had claimed by doing Reiki, remembering the principles, asking Spirit for help, and listening to the guidance she had received. She had learned "the secret method of inviting happiness."

My friend, Reiki master and intuitive reader Linda Urie, says that no one is happy all the time. Everyone has some difficulties and faces some crises. Otherwise, how would we grow? The challenges that confront us stimulate us to become more mindful of our thoughts and feelings so that we can choose to think and behave in more positive ways. This enables us to accept and embrace change.

"A happy life is like a string of pearls," she says, "one happy moment after another, all strung together in a row. Someone who lives a truly happy life experiences many, many happy moments, not constant happiness—but the end result is beautiful, stunning." Her advice to anyone who wants to be happy is to aim to be happy one moment at a time, moment after moment, "just for today."

A WALK IN BEAUTY

Paula Heller lives on a patch of old Pennsylvania farmland, backed by woods and fronted by a stream, a tributary of the Perkiomen Creek, which flows into the Schuylkill River, which joins the Delaware River on its way to the Atlantic Ocean. On a June evening, several Reiki friends gathered in front of her farmhouse around a "fire" of four citronella candles to do Reiki earth healing.

Paula explained: "The land feels sad. There's a meadow that borders the woods, and I believe there was an Indian encampment there. And they were attacked; they were massacred. The land absorbed their blood and sorrow.

"And there's something wrong with the water. There are fish, but there are no frogs. Where have they all gone? And listen! Where are the crickets? Where have they gone? The woods are silent."

We sent Reiki distant healing and asked for guidance. Each of us had something to contribute to the ceremony, some part of the vision to present. We saw the problem not only as the land's memory of atrocity, of man's inhumanity to man, but also as a response to the nearby factory that drains its industrial waste into the creek. Of course, the factory waste complies with federal environmental regulations, but the land and water still seemed to be slowly dying.

"We are to open up the land to joy," Anna said.

Karen Thompson smiled at this remark and asked, "Did you see the fireflies?" Some of us nodded. As she sent Reiki, fireflies came and walked over her fingers and flew between her palms, making her hands glow as if lit from within.

Anna asked me if I had a sense of what to do next. I offered a Reiki healing meditation that I had practiced for several months, adapting it for the earth healing we were there to do. "Lift up your hands and hold them out, palms up.

Call in this land as it is, wounded, onto the palm of your left hand. Now call in this land, as it might be in health and balance, onto the palm of your right hand. Offer Reiki for the highest good and visualize the distant-healing symbols between, bringing healing to both the past and future, and energizing the path between them so that it's easier to travel. Feel the energy flow. You'll feel the energy shift when you're done."

We did this meditation, first with the woodlands and the meadow, then with the millstream and the pond. Our hands tingled, our fingertips sang energy into the earth, our faces shone golden in the candlelight, and we all smiled. On this particular night, we were creating sacred ceremony to bring healing to Mother Earth, and we all felt joy.

Someone asked Paula if she had collected any creek water.

"Yes," she said. "I use it to water the garden. I have some in a bucket and some in a watering can."

"We could charge the water with Reiki and use it to heal the millstream."

"I'll go get it," she said, rising. She returned with a blue bucket, which she placed on the ground among the four candles. We beamed energy at the creek water and then sang.

Karen Biehl, who was trained in opera, led us, chanting the sacred name of the second symbol. We joined in, following her until we knew and could hold the rhythm of the bass line. Then she sang a melody, her voice rising and falling against the bass line on the flow of energy. All around us, the woods, the mill creek and stream, and the meadow we had not yet seen listened—and began to come into harmony.

Our song went on and on until we were interrupted by the lights of a car coming toward us in the driveway and the crunch of gravel under tires as the car pulled to a stop. Like children interrupted, our voices fell into natural silence, as we waited to see who was coming. Paula's son stepped out of the darkness into the light of our circle. He was the one who had created the path we would later walk to the meadow. He had mown and cut a swath a few feet wide, planting low solar lights at intervals so we would be able to see where to step. We thanked him and invited him to join us, but he was content to go inside the house to sleep.

Then we took up our citronella candles and turned on our flashlights, and followed a path through bamboo and brush to the millstream. We stood shoulder to shoulder at one end, looking out over the water in the darkness. We shone flashlights out over its span to see how far it extended. We saw how the trees arched their branches low over the water, as if sheltering it. A bat fluttered into the artificial light, intent on insects.

We put our flashlights and candles down on the ground at our feet, and then raised our hands to send Reiki into the air, water, and land. It seemed absolutely right to use the Reiki symbols, visualizing them on the backs of our hands, blowing them through our hands out over the water, where they would only bring healing.

Paula had carried the bucket of Reiki-charged water with her. Now she dipped her hands into it, cupped them, lifted them out full of "holy water," and poured it into the millstream. We sent more Reiki energy out into the air and water. Without a word, we all knew when our healing ceremony at this place was done.

Next we walked to the meadow, lighting one another's way with flashlights and candles. Once we emerged out of the woods, the full moon, the second one that June, also lit our path. We all sensed when we had come to the place of the massacre, and we all knew we were bringing healing. The midnight sky was clear, the deepest, darkest blue, and dotted with hundreds of stars. We shone our flashlights over the meadow and saw that it was lush with tall grasses and summer wildflowers. We could make out tiny blue flowers at our feet. Fireflies glowed and dimmed, so that the meadow seemed to dance with light, a mirror of the sky. We were all struck silent with wonder: there was so much beauty and harmony there. We felt it within our hearts, as we stood shoulder to shoulder in friendship, a spiritual family.

Again, we set down our flashlights and candles, then stood and faced the meadow, raising our hands to radiate Reiki. None of us knew *how* to bring healing there, to that place where our ancestors in the human family were massacred, but we had all witnessed miracles and trusted the energy. So we offered healing anyway, and as familiar as we were with Reiki, were still surprised when healing came to us. The unity we felt was a fast-acting antidote for every moment of loneliness and isolation each of us had felt in the past. We laughed like children, at home in a meadow full of wildflowers, fireflies, and moonlight, surprised by happiness.

SMALL MIRACLES

Months later, in the early days of cold November, I rescued some of the last nasturtium blossoms from the garden and placed them in a glazed earthenware vase, which I filled with water. Then I held the vase in my hands, feeling the Reiki flow. The next morning, the six blossoms stood as erect as sentinels, their colors bright scarlet, brilliant orange, and glowing yellow.

I was grateful for this small miracle, which reminded me of others, such as the wild phlox that I had gathered and placed in a cut-glass pitcher for a weekend class with some of my Reiki master students. Despite all my previous experience with the fragility and short life span of cut wildflowers, these phlox absorbed the Reiki energy that saturated our classroom. They were sweetly fragrant for days, and their petals didn't fall for almost two weeks. Every day, I admired their delicate beauty and appreciated their astonishing longevity as they sat on my shelf beside a photo of Mikao Usui.

Then I flashed on another small miracle . . .

One summer morning, as I walked, I saw the still form of a swallowtail butterfly at the edge of the asphalt road. I was instantly saddened as I thought of the creature's brief life ending as it flew against a car's windshield. I knelt down beside the motionless body so that I could hold my hands over it. Perhaps by beaming Reiki, I could help the spirit of the butterfly complete its transition.

The draw, which was negligible at first, became stronger. Minutes went by. A truck drove past me and disappeared as it turned onto a side road. Still, the Reiki energy continued to flow. I stayed, wanting to honor the process of healing.

Finally, the energy ebbed. To my astonishment, the butterfly slowly began to flutter its wings, as if waking up from a long nap. I pulled my hands back to make room. Then it lifted up and flew away so abruptly, I was left kneeling on the edge of the road, my eyes wide with sudden tears.

I stood and turned to watch the swallowtail's flight. It raced away in the air, over a field dotted with wildflowers: sun-faced white daisies, bright blue chicory, and the yellow and white snapdragon-like flower called "butter 'n' eggs."

Have I gotten used to miracles? Have I come to expect them? Perhaps I have.

It has been my privilege to join with others in sending Reiki to a man who, though not expected to emerge from a coma, surprised his mother, his doctors, his nurses, and everyone with the question, "Mom, when can I get out of here?" and complete recovery in good humor.

I've witnessed a man who was hunchbacked from years of multiple sclerosis receive Reiki on the bodywork table in a Reiki I class, then get off the table, and stand to his full height of five feet ten inches without even realizing he was doing so.

I've had the pleasure of being informed by one of my students, who began her months of training for certification as a Reiki master with a brain tumor and did nothing but Reiki and refuse to worry, that she was now cancer free. "The brain tumor is gone, and the doctors can't explain it!" she told me, smiling as if she knew a wonderful secret.

Learning to accept that such miracles occur and that, in my life, they're even commonplace has changed me. I no longer accept any medical diagnosis as final. I think of a preliminary diagnosis or early test results as a special window of opportunity for intense, targeted Reiki healing. Although I still occasionally have blue days or hours, I no longer experience depression. I remain calm and usually feel content. I trust in the energy and in Spirit with a positive expectation, a joyful knowing that accompanies happiness.

This is not to say that I don't have challenges in my life. I do, just as every human being does. Some of the challenges that I experience are at the Reiki table or in the classroom, which is as it should be. Like every other practitioner and teacher, I'm meant to grow in my understanding of Reiki. When I first experienced the touch of invisible hands giving me healing, I felt challenged. When a ghost dropped in to observe a Reiki class, I had to keep reminding myself "just for today, do not worry." When I received a Reiki treatment and felt the sensations of a full blood cleanse, hearing every beat of my heart, feeling every surge of blood circulating through my body, I felt right at the limit of my comfort zone. I recognize that sometimes, to help me heal and grow, Reiki invites me to extend my trust further than I have before. When I do, I'm rewarded with a deeper knowledge of the nature of the energy and its source in Spirit.

ONE OF
HAWAYO TAKATA'S MIRACLES

Often, I think about a story Reiki Master Beth Gray told her students about her own teacher, Hawayo Takata. One day, Takata heard a knock on her door. She opened it to a student whose eyes were full of sadness. "Mother has died," the student said. "Would you please return with me to the house, while the family meets to discuss funeral arrangements? We would like you to sit with our mother."

Takata could not refuse such a request. She accompanied the student home and went into the bedroom, where the woman's body was laid out on the bed, as still and cold as death. Takata did not know what to do, except Reiki. She pulled a chair up to the bedside and took the woman's lifeless hand in her own. She felt the gentle current of the energy's flow and prayed for the woman's soul.

After a time, she said to herself, "Well, the woman's hand does not seem quite so cold anymore. Perhaps that is just the Reiki warming her hand." And she continued to give the woman Reiki.

An hour or so went by, and most of the time, Takata had her eyes closed, but when she did open them, she said to herself, "This woman does not look so bad now. There is even a bit of color in her cheeks." Then Takata's eyes drifted closed again, as she continued giving the woman Reiki.

Then several things happened at once. The door opened. Takata looked up to see who had come. The woman on the bed opened her eyes and said, "Oh, I am *so* hungry! Get me some noodles, please!"

Takata, who still held the woman's hand, saw that her student, who stood just inside the door, was stunned with shock. "You heard your mother!" she ordered. "She is hungry! Please get her some noodles."

Even though I heard Reiki Master Beth Gray tell this story several times during the dozen or so classes at which I assisted between 1987 and her retirement from teaching in 1992, I thought it scarcely creditable. I rejected it. I thought that it had to be an exaggeration. Could Reiki raise the dead? Please!

Because I could not consciously accept the story, I repressed the memory of its telling.

About ten years later, after I had taught for a few years and my own experiences with Reiki had begun to seem, at times, miraculous, one of my students gave me a gift, an audiocassette called *Takata Speaks*. This tape was a compilation of stories Hawayo Takata told during classes and talks in the Grays' home in California in the 1970s; it was recorded with Takata's knowledge and permission. As I listened to the tape, I was surprised to hear the story of the woman who was brought back to life by Reiki. Whether or not I could accept the story with my conscious mind, there was Takata's voice, telling the story for me to hear once more and claiming it as truth.

THE POWER OF
REIKI HANDS JOINED IN HEALING

Recently, I taught a Reiki I class to nine students. One of them was a gentleman named Kenneth Donnelly. He and his partner, who was also a student at the class, showed up at the next Reikishare. They had gone out shopping that morning and bought a bodywork table. Both were very excited about learning Reiki and anxious to get started doing treatments.

The following month, Ken came to the Reikishare again and told everyone this story: "Yesterday, the most amazing thing happened to me. I was with a friend at a holistic fair in York. We visited a tent where practitioners working in several different modalities offered mini-sessions. My friend was having her feet massaged, while I waited in line for a psychic reading.

"Suddenly, this older man collapsed. He'd been sitting in a chair at a table, and all of a sudden, he just slumped over and fell onto the floor. Someone called 911 right away, of course, but from all over the tent, Reiki practitioners came forward. A half dozen of us knelt down around him, and we all started beaming Reiki. He was very pale and still, and he wasn't breathing.

"The energy was really intense, and we kept beaming it to him for several minutes. Then he gasped. He took in this huge lungful of air and started breathing normally again. This was about eight or nine minutes after he had collapsed. The paramedics got there right after that.

"I felt so much awe that the Reiki energy could do that, and I feel so grateful to have been there for him and to have had this experience."

Everyone at the Reikishare smiled at Ken. We were all glad for him. "I think you've just had your first Reiki miracle," I told him, "and it's a big one!"

He grinned. "There will be more miracles?"

I nodded. Then I shared Takata's story about using Reiki on a woman who was dead. I reminded him, "Reiki will never interfere with the will of the soul, but sometimes, yes, there are miracles! Mikao Usui called Reiki 'The Secret Method of Inviting Happiness' and 'The Miracle Medicine for All Diseases.' There will be more miracles. Reiki is a path of miracles."

It is a great blessing to learn Reiki. It is so simple, so gentle, so transforming. It invites us to step onto a spiritual path that promises great fulfillment: health, well-being, and happiness. Mikao Usui gave us not only Reiki natural healing but also the Reiki principles to guide us during our daily lives: just for today, do not anger, do not worry, be grateful, do an honest day's work, and be kind. It is up to us to accept the invitation to happiness that he hands to us. Meditate on the Reiki principles. Live the values of peace, serenity, gratitude, integrity, and kindness. Discover the light of wisdom that they shine on the path of life.

SUMMARY

The Reiki principles in their complete form, with the double titles and the recommendation to meditate, are like a spiritual treasure map. Is daily recitation of the principles and mindfulness of the values they express a secret way to invite happiness into our lives? Or does this spiritual practice unlock the gates of the Reiki energy so that we feel even more intense sensations in our hands and experience more and more miracles? What is the relationship between remembering the principles and experiencing the energy? In his own hand, Mikao Usui painted the gentle brushstrokes on rice paper, leaving a puzzle to his followers for many generations to come, an invitation to happiness, and a promise of miracles.

Like learning to listen to the energy, learning to be mindful of the principles calls for an inward focus and attention. By listening to the energy as it flows through our hands, we learn much about the nature of true healing and its source in Spirit; we also learn about our own connection to Spirit and our essential nature. Being mindful of the principles teaches us similar lessons. The principles offer for contemplation the same qualities the energy expresses as it flows through our hands to bring healing: peace, calmness and serenity, gratitude, integrity, and kindness. These are the qualities of the soul awakened by Spirit through Reiki practice, revealing the light and enduring essence of our nature.

MORE SUGGESTIONS FOR PRACTICE

✤ Find an image you like of the Japanese text of the complete Reiki principles. Frame and hang it where you will see it at sunrise. Or you might use an upright-standing frame and place it on your altar, which can be as simple as a single bookshelf or the top of a chest of drawers. Keep the area clean, and make it beautiful and appealing so you will be drawn to it often. When you visit your altar, let yourself become more mindful of the principles.

✤ Commit to reciting the principles twice each day, morning and night, as Mikao Usui suggested. Perhaps you do hands-on healing before getting out of bed in the morning and as you fall asleep at night. If so, recalling the principles at these times creates a gentle transition from sleep to wakefulness and from wakefulness to sleep, and also establishes intention. If this seems too informal, create your own ritual that begins with your hands in gassho and continues in a way that feels right to you.

✤ One way to become more familiar with the subtlety of a language is to learn to speak it well. While becoming fluent in Japanese is an enormous challenge, there are books and tapes that present the pronunciation of the Reiki principles in Japanese. If it feels appropriate and right for you to familiarize yourself with the original language in which the principles were presented, do some online research to discover possible resources. The double VHS tape *Japanese Reiki Techniques Workshop* by Frank Arjava Petter and Chetna Kobayashi will allow you to hear the Japanese pronounced. Some books also present the principles with both an English translation and accompanying Japanese words, which can be read aloud. These include Dave King's *O-Sensei: A View of Mikao Usui*[2] and Frank Arjava Petter's book *Reiki: The Legacy of Dr. Usui*.[3]

❧ Another aid to knowing the power something holds is to trace it with your own hand, as all advanced Reiki practitioners and teachers know well from learning the Reiki symbols and feeling the energy focused through them for various healing purposes. If you are truly ambitious, you may want to learn Japanese calligraphy so you can make the brushstrokes of each ideogram of the principles in your own hand, noticing the energy as you do. When you have finished, take a few minutes to become quiet and listen within. What is the impact of this exercise? Did you feel yourself set aside impatience and frustration as you steadied your brush, stroke after stroke? Did you allow yourself to let go of any mistakes, along with worry? Did you feel a sense of gratitude as the principles emerged at the tip of your brush? In Japan, it is common to look upon art and calligraphy as spiritual pathwork. If you are satisfied with your efforts, both the external expression and the inner awareness, frame the document you have created and place it where you can enjoy it as a reminder of the value of the principles in your life. If you are dissatisfied with your efforts, return to the task another day in the spirit of meditation.

❧ In a lighter vein, help yourself to remember the principles by handwriting them in English or typing and printing them out in a font that appeals to you. Make a visual collage of images that remind you of the values expressed in the principles, let it serve as a background or mat, and then frame your work. Or if you prefer, create a simple border for the principles that will remind you that they help your spiritual pathwork.

❧ One of my Reiki master friends asks her level III students to create their own meditations for each of the principles. She encourages them to do this, not only to prepare them to present the principles in their Reiki I classes but also to help them consider each of the principles more deeply. She invites them to take weeks to think about each principle and then write something to share with the class. If you are tempted to undertake such a task, listen to the energy for guidance. Be assured that making a sincere effort to understand and appreciate the values the principles express will move you forward on the Reiki path in new and wonderful ways. There is deep satisfaction in this soul work, for it brings illumination as well as moments of joy, peace, and contentment. This is happiness "just for today."

Epilogue

THE SPIRAL PATH

Have you ever held a nautilus shell in your hand and traced its gentle curve as it arced inward to its center? Have you noticed the pale delicacy of the shell's colors as they change and deepen near the heart? Have you let your eye retrace the curve, the pathway the sea creature must travel when it ventures forward? The shell is shelter and pathway, the nautilus's world and its way in the world.

The spiral of the first symbol marks a pathway. It is the pathway of the energy itself as it enters us from above and radiates out in widening circles, the pathway of the energy through the symbol as we draw it to call for healing, and the journey of life entered into at birth and traveled with increasing awareness to journey's end. The Reiki principles, too, offer us a pathway, a journey that we can take in a moment and travel moment by moment, as pathwork, over the course of a lifetime.

When we refuse to anger, we hold in or hold back the intense energy of that negative emotion. We withdraw or retreat within. When we refuse to worry or become anxious, we check the impulse to scatter energy in negative emotion. We shift our attention away from whatever provokes us and focus on the feeling of the energy, remembrance of the principles, the movement of our own breath, and the consciousness of peace within. In that awareness of inner peace, we find sanctuary. Gratitude fills us. We are renewed. We choose to focus our energy in positive ways. We do our best. We are kind. We have traveled the spiral pathway, withdrawing to center and expanding from center. The Reiki principles guide us within, support and strengthen us, and then encourage us to reenter the world with grace and wisdom; as shelter and pathway, they show us a way of being in the world.

WALKING THE PATH, DAY BY DAY

A recently certified Reiki master phoned me one evening to talk about a problem. "When I do distant healing on myself," she said, "I keep seeing an image of Jesus. I grew up Jewish, and I find this really disturbing. What do you think this is about?"

"How does this image make you feel?"

"Well, it makes me feel angry, I guess. I'm not necessarily angry at Christ, but I do feel angry that Christians have persecuted Jews during most of the last two thousand years."

"So is it possible that this image is making you more aware of an issue that needs some healing?"

"Yes, I guess so." She sighed, releasing some of her frustration. "Have you ever seen an image of Jesus as you did Reiki?"

"Yes, and I've also seen Buddha, Krishna, and others who were beloved as enlightened beings and spiritual teachers."

"And you're okay with it?"

"Yes, I welcome such impressions as a sign of blessings."

"I've seen Buddha several times before, but it never bothered me. I guess I have very different feelings about Christianity than Buddhism. I had relatives who were sent to concentration camps and died in the Holocaust, and I think most members of the Jewish community share this experience. I also get angry when I hear anti-Semitic comments or read stories about swastikas in the news. It seems like there are still a lot of negative attitudes hidden under the surface. So when I see Jesus, I associate that with anti-Semitic hatred."

"I understand that."

"So I'm just going to have to work on healing this anger?"

"I think so. It would be good to work toward forgiveness and tolerance."

"So I send Reiki to heal my inability to forgive?"

"That might be a good place to start—and remember to let go of your anger 'just for today.'"

The day I visited Iryna Zhyrenko to interview her about her journey to the United States from the Ukraine, she confided to me that she was very worried about a numbness she had felt in her right arm. She had experienced several episodes over the past week and a half. She had visited her doctor, and because she had also experienced migraines, he was concerned as well. He ordered further diagnostic tests to rule out a brain tumor. She was frightened for her son and herself.

She asked me if I would attune her, even though she knew that she didn't need to be re-attuned. She wanted the healing that the attunement would bring. She admitted that, besides feeling concerned about this unknown medical problem, she was very stressed out about her job. Since coming to the United States six years ago, she had been granted a divorce, become naturalized as a citizen, and graduated with a master's degree in counseling psychology. Now she worked in a counseling center for drug and alcohol addiction but she found it a depressing atmosphere.

"I don't feel my hands so strongly now," she complained. "I don't know what's wrong."

"How much have you been practicing?"

"Not so much. Not enough," she admitted. "I need to practice more."

I agreed to attune her, so she found a comfortable chair, sat down, and placed her hands in gassho. I bowed to her and began the attunement, focusing on the energy, the symbols, and the steps.

Afterward, she gave me a dazzling smile and said, "Thank you so much. I really felt a shift. I feel better, lighter!"

"You're welcome. Thank you for being willing to let me interview you." I gathered my notebook and purse, gave her a hug, and left.

Two days later, she called me. "Something happened after the attunement!" she said. "You remember that I was so frightened about the numbness?"

"Yes."

"A couple of hours after the attunement, both my arms went numb. I went to the emergency room, and the doctor took X-rays. Guess what? No brain tumor! The vertebrae in my neck were out of alignment and pressed on the nerves, causing the numbness down my arms. So an orthopedic doctor in the emergency room did an adjustment. The numbness is gone! I am fine!"

"That Reiki attunement did bring you healing."

"Oh, yes!"

I thought about other experiences I'd had when the Reiki energy healed by bringing the true nature of a medical condition to light. This resulted in changes in medication and diagnosis. It occurred to me that this was one more way the energy reinforces the message of the Reiki principles, so I reminded Iryna of this.

"Yes, yes! 'Just for today, do not worry.' I will remember this."

"I feel so fortunate," Mike Sebio said, while sitting in a circle with other Reiki master students. "I have a wonderful wife. I love my daughter. Now I have two wonderful grandchildren." He paused, his eyes unfocused as he pondered his life. The expression on his face was almost tender. He continued, "I have a good job as a manager of computer operations. It's a demanding job but a good one. Because of it, our house is paid for. Now I'm looking forward to retirement, when I'll have more time to be with my family and to do Reiki."

He was back with us, alert and smiling. His appreciation for all the blessings in his life touched us. He had so much humility. I imagined him quietly telling his clients that he didn't regard himself as a healer, that the energy was the healer. Several of his clients had recently expressed the desire to have him teach them Reiki, but he had to wait until I certified him, a process that would take months; yet he wasn't impatient. He was staying the course and enjoying the shelter of gratitude.

At the end of November 2007, Beverly Schultz, a newly initiated Reiki master, wrote to me asking how I teach the history of Reiki:

I am preparing to begin teaching Reiki, and as I gather my materials, I realize there is so much more information regarding the history of Reiki than when I first learned. My heart tells me to stay with the traditional story of the beginning of Reiki . . . I guess I am asking you what you think of staying with the traditional story and noting that research is finding new information about the origin. I think I just answered my question but would love your thoughts.[1]

Every Reiki master is challenged to teach Reiki with integrity. This means that we must be willing to honor the tradition or traditions in which we were taught and also our personal experiences with the energy. This creates some interesting dilemmas, as new, documented information becomes available to us. When it comes to the history of Reiki, I am pleased to pass along Takata's story, which I value for its wisdom, insight, and beautiful, parable-like form. I am also glad to share what I have learned about Mikao Usui's life from the translations of the inscription on his memorial outside Saihoji Temple in Tokyo. Why would I not be glad to share whatever information I have? Yet I know that history does not present essential spiritual truth in the same way that simply doing Reiki does.

Reiki invites us all to draw healing from the same Source. If we continue to practice, we will learn about the nature of that Source, and this brings spiritual healing to us all so that eventually we come to a sense of wholeness, spiritual integrity, and community. When I teach a class, I tell my students, as I was told, "Reiki is the healer," but I also add, "Reiki is the teacher." The best way to learn Reiki is to practice. Since Reiki is experiential, we learn more about what is true of Reiki from practice than in any other way.

The ongoing preoccupation that many Reiki masters have with the question of integrity is a blessing. Because we are involved with Reiki in a dynamic, vital learning process, we become more willing to look at every aspect of our lives with active attention and engagement. While Reiki practitioners may not be challenged to speak about the truth of their experiences with Reiki as often as Reiki teachers, they, too, search for words that will describe the sensations they feel in their hands, the healing they witness, and the quiet joy that awakens in their hearts.

"Would you like me to get your table for you, Amy?" Jim Chokas offered.

I grinned up at him. He was a big man, maybe six feet three, and broad-shouldered with muscles. "You know I would."

He laughed and shrugged. "I just thought I would ask."

"Thank you! You have perfect timing. Here are the car keys, and here's the key to the trunk."

He hefted the black case by the strap onto his shoulder as if it weighed nothing. "I'll see you at your car," he said, turning toward the door.

As it shut behind him, I thought, *Reiki practitioners and teachers are the kindest people I know. Over and over again, they are kind. It comes to them as naturally as breathing. They think of others, consider their needs, offer to help when unasked, and help willingly when asked. They do practice the principle "Just for today, be kind."*

Reiki Master Ellen Philips recites the Reiki principles each morning without fail. In a workshop on the Reiki principles that we co-taught, she joked that she had found the perfect way to remember them. She had printed out an English translation she liked and placed it on her refrigerator, beneath photos of Mikao Usui, Chujiro Hayashi, and Hawayo Takata. This way, every time she goes to the refrigerator, she is reminded of the Reiki principles!

Despite her sense of humor about this practice, she is serious in her intention to follow Mikao Usui's recommendation to recite the principles morning and night. Each morning, as soon as she gets out of bed, brushes her teeth, and goes into the kitchen, she stands before the principles and the photos of the early teachers, brings her hands together in gassho, bows, and feels her heart expand with gratitude for Reiki. Then she recites the principles, slowly and thoughtfully. As a result, throughout the day, she remains mindful of the values they express.

DAILY PRACTICE, DAILY REMEMBRANCE

We can make considerable progress on the path of Reiki simply by doing energy healing. When we claim that strong, clear connection to Spirit that comes through doing Reiki, we generally manifest more of our spiritual nature: we radiate peace, feel calm and serene, readily appreciate the good in our lives, aspire to excellence and work toward it with integrity, and find many ways to be kind. This enhances the overall quality of our lives, making it easier for us to feel content and happy. We may even find that we have attracted some greater good.

Sooner or later, however, we will be faced with a difficulty, challenge, or crisis; find ourselves involved with others who have problems; or remember an issue that still needs healing. During such times, even if we remain steadfast in our commitment to do Reiki each day, happiness is likely to seem fleeting unless we make the additional effort to live by the principles. The principles become invaluable tools for claiming—and reclaiming—health, well-being, and happiness. When we adopt them and allow ourselves to be guided by them, we bring healing into the world in another way.

When we control the impulse to react in anger or quiet anxious thoughts, we calm fear-based feelings "just for today." This discipline requires an act of will, but it may also be performed as an act of love that arises from self-knowledge, devotion, and wisdom. The refusal to anger or to be anxious sets our feet once more on the spiritual path. Standing centered in the awareness that we are showered with blessings, we are cleansed of negativity. Positive thoughts and feelings flood us. Steadied and strengthened, we move forward again with grace and ease. Now we respond to challenge and confrontation guided by the best impulses of our being. We are inspired, we perform well, we produce work of the highest quality, and we do so with graciousness and generosity. We radiate love into our world. We light the way for others to follow, even as we make out the next steps we are to take, just ahead. This, too, is a way of listening to the energy.

As we listen to the energy as we do hands-on and distant healing, we learn about the nature and source of healing; over time, we gradually come to understand that we are learning about our own essential nature and its origin in Spirit. Practicing the Reiki principles invites us to learn the same lessons in the school of life. We need not choose between energy healing and the principles as spiritual pathwork, for they teach and reinforce the same lessons. When we integrate and understand these lessons, our lives become illumined by the

233

awareness of the values Reiki teaches: peace, serenity, appreciation, integrity and wholeness, kindness. We begin to understand that greater healing than we have ever imagined is possible in this world—and isn't that a happy thought?

Mikao Usui's experiences on Mt. Kurama changed him from a man seeking enlightenment to a man who sought to serve humanity. His spontaneous attunement enabled him to share with humanity the great spiritual gifts that he had received. Now, generations of people have received healing through Reiki and experienced its power to transform their lives in countless positive ways. Remembrance of the principles, which Mikao Usui thought so important, is not only a way to bring healing into the world; it is a way to honor him, and it is a way to express our gratitude to Spirit. The energy is the healer, but we may make the effort to align our individual consciousness with the purpose of healing out of love for the energy. In this way, too, as we walk the path of Reiki, we may join with others around the world to contribute to world healing and peace.

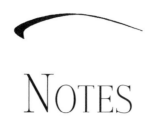

NOTES

CHAPTER 1. THE PATH OF REIKI

1. Lauren Bissett, private correspondence (April 3, 2005).

2. Hiroshi Doi, "Usui Reiki Ryoho International Workshop 2002" (lecture and conference proceedings [Saturday 30–31], Toronto, Canada, September 28, 2002).

3. Although the presentation here follows my sense of the techniques, I have referred back to my class notes and the manual I was given during my training with Tom Rigler on April 20 and 21, 2001, for details. In addition, I have consulted the conference proceedings from the "Usui Reiki Ryoho International Workshop" presented in Toronto, Canada, September 27–29, 2002. Hiroshi Doi shared this technique with the Reiki masters gathered on September 28, 2002, with the encouragement to relay the information to our students.

CHAPTER 2. THE REIKI PRINCIPLES

1. Helen Haberly, *Reiki: Hawayo Takata's Story* (Olney, MD: Archedigm, 1990), 8.

2. Fran Brown, *Living Reiki: Takata's Teachings* (Mendocino, CA: Life Rhythm, 1992), 52.

3. Anneli Twan, *Early Days of Reiki: Memories of Hawayo Takata* (Hope, BC, Canada: Morning Star Productions, 2005), 14.

4. Frank Arjava Petter, *Reiki Fire: New Information about the Origins of the Reiki Power; A Complete Manual* (Twin Lakes, WI: Lotus Light Publications, 1997), 23.

5. Hiroshi Doi, "Usui Reiki Ryoho International Workshop 2002" (lecture and conference proceedings [Saturday 3], Toronto, Canada, September 28, 2002).

6. Frank Arjava Petter, *Reiki Fire: New Information about the Origins of the Reiki*

Power; A Complete Manual (Twin Lakes, WI: Lotus Light Publications, 1997), 30.

7. Ibid., 22.

8. Ibid., 23.

9. Frank Arjava Petter, *Reiki: The Legacy of Dr. Usui* (Twin Lakes, WI: Lotus Light Publications, 1998), 29.

10. Andrew Bowling, foreword to *Iyashino Gendai Reiki-ho: Modern Reiki Method for Healing,* by Hiroshi Doi, edited by Rick Rivard and Miyuki Iwasaki, translated by Akiko Kawarai, Mari Marchand, Hiroko and Phillip Kelly, Emiko Arai, Yukio Miura, and Yuko Okamoto (Coquitlam, BC, Canada: Fraser, 2000), 4.

11. Hiroshi Doi, *Iyashino Gendai Reiki-ho: Modern Reiki Method for Healing,* edited by Rick Rivard and Miyuki Iwasaki, translated by Akiko Kawarai, Mari Marchand, Hiroko and Phillip Kelly, Emiko Arai, Yukio Miura, and Yuko Okamoto (Coquitlam, BC, Canada: Fraser, 2000), 131–32.

12. Ibid., 129.

13. Bronwen and Frans Stiene, *The Reiki Sourcebook* (Hants, UK: O Books, 2003), appendix D, 349–51.

14. Hiroshi Doi, "Usui Reiki Ryoho International Workshop 2002" (lecture, Toronto, Canada, September 28, 2002).

15. Hyakuten Inamoto, *Komyo Reiki Kai: Reiki Healing Art* (Kyoto, Japan: Komyo Reiki Kai, 2002), 24.

16. Dave King, *O-Sensei: A View of Mikao Usui* (Morrisville, NC: Dave King/Lulu, 2006; available at www.book.usui-do.org), 6.

17. Ibid., 31.

18. Ibid., 32.

CHAPTER 3. PEACE:
"JUST FOR TODAY, DO NOT ANGER"

1. Fran Brown, *Living Reiki: Takata's Teachings* (Mendocino, CA: Life Rhythm, 1992), 94.

2. Ibid., 38.

CHAPTER 4. SERENITY:
"JUST FOR TODAY, DO NOT WORRY"

1. Fran Brown, *Living Reiki: Takata's Teachings* (Mendocino, CA: Life Rhythm, 1992), 19.

2. Ibid.

3. Hiroshi Doi, "Usui Reiki Ryoho International Workshop 2002" (lecture and conference proceedings [Saturday 32], Toronto, Canada, September 28, 2002).

4. Frank Arjava Petter, *Reiki Fire: New Information about the Origins of the Reiki Power; A Complete Manual* (Twin Lakes, WI: Lotus Light Publications, 1997), 31.

CHAPTER 5. GRATITUDE:
"BE GRATEFUL: SHOW APPRECIATION"

1. Hawayo Takata, in "Extracts from Takata-Sensei's Diaries 1935/1936" (www .aetw.org/reiki_takata_diary.htm, accessed May 12, 2008).

2. Aimee Kovac, private correspondence (June 5, 2007).

3. Sarah Ban Breathnach, *Simple Abundance: A Daybook of Comfort and Joy* (New York: Warner Books, Inc., 1995).

CHAPTER 6. INTEGRITY:
"DO AN HONEST DAY'S WORK"

1. Frank Arjava Petter, *Reiki Fire: New Information about the Origins of the Reiki Power; A Complete Manual* (Twin Lakes, WI: Lotus Light Publications, 1997).

2. Frank Arjava Petter, *Reiki: The Legacy of Dr. Usui* (Twin Lakes, WI: Lotus Light Publications, 1998).

3. Hiroshi Doi, "Usui Reiki Ryoho International Workshop 2002" (lecture and conference proceedings [Saturday 32], Toronto, Canada, September 28, 2002).

4. Ibid.

5. Hiroshi Doi, "Usui Reiki Ryoho International Workshop 2002" (lecture, Toronto, Canada, September 27–29, 2002).

6. Fran Brown, *Living Reiki: Takata's Teachings* (Mendocino, CA: Life Rhythm, 1992), 58–59.

7. Helen Haberly, *Reiki: Hawayo Takata's Story* (Olney, MD: Archedigm, 1990), 38–42.

8. Fran Brown, *Living Reiki: Takata's Teachings* (Mendocino, CA: Life Rhythm, 1992), 59.

9. Eckhart Tolle, *A New Earth: Awakening to Your Life's Purpose* (New York: Dutton/Penguin Group, Inc., 2005), 95.

CHAPTER 7. KINDNESS:
"BE KIND"

1. Hiroshi Doi, "Usui Reiki Ryoho International Workshop 2002" (lecture, Toronto, Canada, September 28, 2002).
2. Frank Arjava Petter, *Reiki Fire: New Information about the Origins of the Reiki Power; A Complete Manual* (Twin Lakes, WI: Lotus Light Publications, 1997), 30.

CHAPTER 8. THE DOUBLE TITLE: AN INVITATION
TO HAPPINESS AND A PROMISE OF MIRACLES

1. Hiroshi Doi, "Usui Reiki Ryoho International Workshop 2002" (lecture, Toronto, Canada, September 28, 2002).
2. Dave King, *O-Sensei: A View of Mikao Usui* (Morrisville, NC: Dave King/Lulu, 2006; available at www.book.usui-do.org), 43–47.
3. Frank Arjava Petter, *Reiki: The Legacy of Dr. Usui* (Twin Lakes, WI: Lotus Light Publications, 1998), 29.

EPILOGUE: THE SPIRAL PATH

1. Beverly Schultz, private correspondence (November 10, 2007).

RECOMMENDED
READING AND LISTENING

ON REIKI

Brown, Fran. *Living Reiki: Takata's Teachings.* Mendocino, CA: Life Rhythm, 1992.

Doi, Hiroshi. *Iyashino Gendai Reiki-ho: Modern Reiki Method for Healing.* Edited by Rick Rivard and Miyuki Iwasaki. Translated by Akiko Kawarai Mari Marchand, Hiroko and Phillip Kelly, Emiko Arai, Yukio Miura, Yuko Okamoto. Coquitlam, BC, Canada: Fraser, 2000.

Gray, John Harvey, and Lourdes Gray, with Steven McFadden and Elisabeth Clark. *Hand to Hand: The Longest-Practicing Reiki Master Tells His Story.* Philadelphia, PA: Xlibris Corporation at www.xlibris.com, 2002.

Haberly, Helen. *Reiki: Hawayo Takata's Story.* Olney, MD: Archedigm, 1990.

Hall, Mari. *Reiki for the Soul: Ten Doorways to Inner Peace.* London: Thorsons Publishers, 2002.

———. *Reiki for the Soul: The Eleventh Doorway.* Sedona, AZ: Infinite Light Healing Studies Center, Inc., 2006.

Honervogt, Tanmaya. *Reiki for Emotional Healing.* London: Gaia Books, 2006.

King, Dave. *O-Sensei: A View of Mikao Usui.* Morrisville, NC: Dave King/Lulu, 2006 (available at www.book.usui-do.org).

Klinger-Omenka, Ursula. *Reiki with Gemstones.* Twin Lakes, WI: Lotus Light Publications, 1997.

Lübeck, Walter, Frank Arjava Petter, and William Lee Rand. *The Spirit of Reiki: The Complete Handbook of the Reiki System.* Twin Lakes, WI: Lotus Press/Shangri-La, 2001.

Miles, Pamela. *Reiki: A Comprehensive Guide*. New York: Penguin Group, 2006.

Petter, Frank Arjava. *Reiki Fire: New Information about the Origins of the Reiki Power; A Complete Manual*. Twin Lakes, WI: Lotus Light Publications/Shangri-La, 1997.

———. *Reiki: The Legacy of Dr. Usui*. Twin Lakes, WI: Lotus Light Publications/Shangri-La, 1998.

Petter, Frank Arjava, and Chetna Kobayashi. *Japanese Reiki Techniques Workshop*. VHS recording. Southfield, MI: Vision Publications, 2000.

Petter, Frank Arjava, Tadao Yamaguchi, and Chujiro Hayashi. *Hayashi Reiki Manual: Traditional Japanese Reiki Healing Techniques from the Founder of the Western Reiki System*. Twin Lakes, WI: Lotus Press/Shangri-La, 2003.

Rand, William Lee. *Reiki for a New Millenium*. New Delhi, India: Health Harmony, 2000.

Rowland, Amy Z. *Traditional Reiki for Our Times: Practical Methods for Personal and Planetary Healing*. Rochester, VT: Healing Arts Press, 1998.

———. *Intuitive Reiki for Our Times: Essential Techniques for Enhancing Your Practice*. Rochester, VT: Healing Arts Press, 2006.

Stiene, Bronwen and Frans. *The Reiki Sourcebook*. Alresford, Hampshire, UK: O Books, 2003.

Takata, Hawayo. *Takata Speaks, Vol. 1: Reiki Stories*. Audiotape of Reiki master training classes conducted in 1976. Rindge, NH: The John Harvey Gray Center for Reiki Healing, n.d.

Twan, Anneli. *Early Days of Reiki: Memories of Hawayo Takata*. Hope, BC, Canada: Morning Star Productions, 2005.

Usui, Mikao, and Frank Arjava Petter. *The Original Reiki Handbook of Dr. Mikao Usui*. Translated by Christine M. Grimm. Twin Lakes, WI: Lotus Press/Shangri-La, 1999.

ON SPIRITUAL PATHWORK

Kabat-Zinn, Jon. *Arriving at Your Own Door: 108 Lessons in Mindfulness*. New York: Hyperion, 2007.

———. *Mindfulness for Beginners*. Boulder, CO: Sounds True, 2006. Two compact discs.

Kornfield, Jack. *Meditation for Beginners*. Boulder, CO: Sounds True, 2001. Two compact discs.

Kurtz, Ernest, and Katherine Ketcham. *The Spirituality of Imperfection: Storytelling and the Journey to Wholeness*. New York: Bantam Books, 1992.

Tolle, Eckhart. *The Power of Now: A Guide to Spiritual Enlightenment*. Novato, CA: New World Library, 2004.

ON HEALING ANGER

Beattie, Melody. *Beyond Codependency: And Getting Better All the Time*. Center City, MN: Hazelden Foundation, 1989.

———. *Codependent No More: How to Stop Controlling Others and Start Caring for Yourself*. Center City, MN: Hazelden Foundation, 1992.

Bradshaw, John. *Homecoming: Reclaiming and Championing Your Inner Child*. New York: Bantam Books, 1990.

Carter, Les. *The Anger Trap: Free Yourself from the Frustrations That Sabotage Your Life*. San Francisco: Jossey-Bass/John Wiley & Sons, 2003.

Chapman, Gary. *Anger: Handling a Powerful Emotion in a Healthy Way*. Chicago: Northfield Publishing, 2007.

Deutschman, Allan. *Change or Die: The Three Keys to Change at Work and in Life*. New York: HarperCollins Publishers, 2007.

Griffin, Kathleen. *The Forgiveness Formula: How to Let Go of Your Pain and Move On with Life*. New York: Marlowe & Company, 2004.

Hanh, Thich Nhat. *Anger: Wisdom for Cooling the Flames*. New York: Riverhead Books, 2001.

Hay, Louise. *You Can Heal Your Life*. Carlsbad, CA: Hay House, Inc., 2004.

———. *Meditations for Personal Healing*. Carlsbad, CA: Hay House, Inc., 2005. Compact disc.

Lerner, Harriet. *The Dance of Anger: A Woman's Guide to Changing the Patterns of Intimate Relationships*. New York: Harper & Row, 1993.

Potter-Efron, Ronald T., and Patricia S. Potter-Efron. *Letting Go of Anger: The Eleven Most Common Anger Styles and What to Do about Them*. Oakland, CA: New Harbinger Publications, 2006.

Progoff, Ira. *At a Journal Workshop: Writing to Access the Power of the Unconscious and Evoke Creative Ability*. New York: Jeremy P. Tarcher/Putnam, 1992.

ON LETTING GO OF WORRY

Brantley, Jeffrey. *Calming Your Anxious Mind: How Mindfulness and Compassion Can Free You from Anxiety, Fear, and Panic.* Oakland, CA: New Harbinger Publications, 2007.

Carnegie, Dale. *How to Stop Worrying and Start Living: Time-Tested Methods for Conquering Worry.* Rev. ed. New York: Pocket Books/Simon & Schuster, 1984.

Chödrön, Pema. *Getting Unstuck: Breaking Your Habitual Patterns and Encountering Naked Reality.* Boulder, CO: Sounds True, 2005. Compact disc.

Day, Laura. *Welcome to Your Crisis: How to Use the Power of Crisis to Create the Life You Want.* New York: Little, Brown and Company, 2006.

Dyer, Wayne W. *There's a Spiritual Solution to Every Problem.* New York: HarperAudio, 2001. Compact disc.

Falcone, Vickie. *Buddha Never Raised Kids and Jesus Didn't Drive Carpool: Seven Principles for Parenting with Soul.* San Diego, CA: Jodere Group, 2003.

Lerner, Harriet. *The Dance of Fear: Rising Above Anxiety, Fear, and Shame to Be Your Best and Bravest Self.* New York: HarperCollins, 2004.

ON GRATITUDE

Braybrooke, Marcus, ed. *The Bridge of Stars: 365 Prayers, Blessings, and Meditations from Around the World.* London: Thorsons Publishers, 2001.

Breathnach, Sarah Ban. *Simple Abundance: A Daybook of Comfort and Joy.* New York: Warner Books, 1995.

DeMartini, John F. *Count Your Blessings: The Healing Power of Gratitude and Love.* Carlsbad, CA: Hay House, 1997, 2006.

Emmons, Robert A. *Thanks! How the New Science of Gratitude Can Make You Happier.* New York: Houghton Mifflin Company, 2007.

Krech, Gregg. *Naikan: Gratitude, Grace, and the Japanese Art of Self-Reflection.* Berkeley, CA: Stone Bridge Press, 2002.

Sark. *Sark's New Creative Companion: Ways to Free Your Creative Spirit.* Berkeley, CA: Celestial Arts, 2005.

ON INTEGRITY

Anthony, Susie. *A Map to God: Awakening Spiritual Integrity.* Winchester, UK: O Books, 2007.

Ruiz, Don Miguel, with Janet Mills. *The Voice of Knowledge: A Practical Guide to Inner Peace.* San Rafael, CA: Amber-Allen Publishing, 2004.

Tolle, Eckhart. *Stillness Speaks.* Novato, CA: New World Library, 2003.

———. *A New Earth: Awakening to Your Life's Purpose.* New York: Plume/Penguin Group, 2006.

ON KINDNESS

Dalai Lama XIV, H. H. *The Spirit of Peace: Teachings on Love, Compassion, and Everyday Life.* London: Thorsons Publishers, 2002.

Ferrucci, Piero. *The Power of Kindness: The Unexpected Benefits of Leading a Compassionate Life.* New York: Jeremy P. Tarcher/Penguin Group, 2006.

Lovasik, Lawrence G. *The Hidden Power of Kindness: A Practical Handbook for Souls Who Dare to Transform the World, One Deed at a Time.* Manchester, NH: Sophia Institute Press, 1999. Abridged ed. of *Kindness* (New York: The MacMillan Company, 1962).

ON HAPPINESS

Ben-Shahar, Tal. *Happier: Learn the Secrets to Daily Joy and Lasting Fulfillment.* New York: McGraw-Hill Books, 2007.

Byrne, Rhonda. *The Secret.* New York: Atria Books, 2006.

Chödrön, Pema. *True Happiness.* Boulder, CO: Sounds True, 2006. 2 Compact discs.

Chopra, Deepak. *Power, Freedom, and Grace: Living from the Source of Lasting Happiness.* San Rafael, CA: Amber-Allen Publishing, 2006.

Csikszentmihalyi, Mihaly. *Flow: The Psychology of Optimal Experience.* New York: HarperCollins Publishers, 1990.

Dalai Lama XIV, H. H., and Howard C. Cutler. *The Art of Happiness: A Handbook for Living.* New York: Riverhead Books/Penguin Group, 1998.

Holden, Robert. *Happiness Now! Timeless Wisdom for Feeling Good Fast.* Carlsbad, CA: Hay House, 2007.

BOOKS OF RELATED INTEREST

Traditional Reiki for Our Times
Practical Methods for Personal and Planetary Healing
by Amy Z. Rowland

Intuitive Reiki for Our Times
Essential Techniques for Enhancing Your Practice
by Amy Z. Rowland

Reiki Energy Medicine
Bringing Healing Touch into Home, Hospital, and Hospice
by Libby Barnett and Maggie Chambers with Susan Davidson

Vibrational Medicine
The #1 Handbook of Subtle-Energy Therapies
by Richard Gerber, M.D.

Accepting Your Power to Heal
The Personal Practice of Therapeutic Touch
by Dolores Krieger, Ph.D., R.N.

Therapeutic Touch Inner Workbook
by Dolores Krieger, Ph.D., R.N.

The Spiritual Dimension of Therapeutic Touch
by Dora Kunz with Dolores Krieger, Ph.D., R.N.

Bodymind Energetics
Toward a Dynamic Model of Health
by Mark Seem, Ph.D., with Joan Kaplan

INNER TRADITIONS • BEAR & COMPANY
P.O. Box 388
Rochester, VT 05767
1-800-246-8648
www.InnerTraditions.com

Or contact your local bookseller